SPIRITUALITY AND MEANING IN HEALTH CARE

Studies in Spirituality Supplements

Edited by

Hein Blommestijn – Kees Waaijman – Frans Maas
Titus Brandsma Institute – Nijmegen – The Netherlands

TITUS BRANDSMA INSTITUTE

STUDIES IN SPIRITUALITY
Supplement 17

SPIRITUALITY AND MEANING IN HEALTH CARE

A Dutch Contribution to an Ongoing Discussion

edited by

J. Bouwer

Translated from the Dutch by Helen-Anne Ross

PEETERS
LEUVEN - PARIS - DUDLEY, MA
2008

A CIP record for this book is available from the Library of Congress.

ISBN 978-90-429-2054-5
D. 2008/0602/40

CONTENTS

J. Bouwer

INTRODUCTION
SPIRITUALITY AND MEANING IN HEALTH CARE

In the Netherlands, increasing attention is paid to the place, the role and the value of spirituality, meaning, and philosophy of life within health care. The occasion for this relates to the place and the function modern medicine occupies in society. As a result of its many victories on various fronts within health care, medicine was implicitly allotted pretensions as to salvation. This has exerted a binding, cementing effect on people who, face to face with illness, suffering, infirmity and death must perforce rely upon it. For health care consumers, pretensions as to salvation have led to an optimism bestowing on medicine a halo of inviolability and sanctity.[1] This has caused the sociologist Ter Borg to state that both world views and the giving of meaning have become medicalised. He argues that it has become necessary to limit medical consumption, by putting the soteriologic import of the medical way of proceeding into perspective.[2]

The place assigned to health care today is symptomatic of other developments and forces in society, which includes health care. The forces of science, economy and technology are virtually ascribed absolute value in our society. They manifest themselves within healthcare as 'evidence-based medicine' and 'managed care'. This implies that rationalisation predominates, translated into a strategy of making 'suitable' use of care that 'should be given at the right moment to the right degree and at the right price on the right grounds', and that moreover should be 'proven effective'.[3] There is an increasing desire to base healthcare on methods founded on research. In addition, the relationship between doctor and patient seems to be ever more regulated by an abundance

---

1 J. Bouwer, *Geestelijke zorgverlening als wetenschappelijke discipline* (Spiritual care provision as scientific discipline), Zeist: CVZ, 1998, 13.

2 M.B. ter Borg, 'Op zoek naar hoop' (Searching for hope), in: M.B. ter Borg, S. van der Geest & J. Janssen, *Op zoek naar hoop: Over genezing, magie en religie* (Searching for hope: About healing, magic and religion), Nijmegen: MacDonald, 1997, 23.

3 D. Post & H. Vermeij, 'De gezondheidszorg als context van de geestelijke verzorging' (Health care as context of spiritual care), in: J.J. Rebel (Ed.), *Wel bezorgd: Geestelijke verzorging en gezondheidszorg* (Well cared for: Spiritual care and health care), Kampen: Kok, 1998, 23.

of healthcare legislation.[4] There is a contract relationship between doctor and patient, whereas this was historically based on a contact conspicuous by its ethics and confidentiality.[5] This relationship is now increasingly influenced by legislation.

Without wishing to shut our eyes to the positive achievements of medicine in recent decades, appeals louder than ever before are being made for an evaluation of the influence these achievements exert on specific human values and characteristics. For the increasing influence of legislation and technology on medicine may pave the wave to dehumanisation.[6] For example, this occurs when persons are objectified and reduced to specific sick but treatable parts. A human being is more than that of course. That is why inquiring into the anthropology supported by those working in care is very topical at the moment. What image of humanity underlies medical and nursing procedure?

In any case, the medicalisation of reality gives rise to the suspicion that a human being is approached solely from the perspective of his biological-physical component in the context of medicine. Various camps resist this one-sidedness. For a human being is a unity within which physical, psychological, social and spiritual aspects can be identified. A holistic vision of humanity argues that good care implies attention to all these components, in relationship to the 'being-ill' of human beings. So attention should also be paid to the spiritual or giving of meaning component of the human being, for an approach to the patient must also consider his experience and needs, set against the background of demand-driven care (new philosophy about care provision). For Ter Borg, the giving of meaning component is therefore essential to attempts to confine medicine's connotation of salvation and put it into perspective.[7]

Western medicine seems to have entered a new era, namely that of so-called holistic medicine, with diverse initiatives being undertaken to view the spiritual component as an integral part of qualitatively good care. The distance that has grown between body and spirit throughout the centuries is being reduced once

[4] D.J. Bakker, 'Het algemene ziekenhuis van onze tijd' (The general hospital of our time), in: *Praktische Theologie* (Practical Theology) 27 (2000), no 4, 372. In this article Bakker analyses the cultural, historical and social context in which the modern hospital finds itself. He concludes among other things that the essentially ethical relationship between doctor and patient may not be replaced with impunity by a legal relationship. He refers to legislation such as the Medical Treatment Agreement Act (WGBO), the Quality Care Institutions Act and the Professions in Individual Healthcare Act (BIG) that are the result of health legislation seeking legal measures in legislation and regulations in favour of the patient. The patient must obtain more rights in the relationship with the doctor which is in unequal in principle.

[5] Ibidem.

[6] Ibid., 373.

[7] Ter Borg, 'Op zoek naar hoop', 33.

more.[8] Advocates of holistic medicine in the United States, where discussion on the integration of religion and spirituality has been raging for some considerable time, refer to Chinese medicine. To this day, a medical intervention in Chinese medicine intends to treat the 'chi' (the energy, life, power or spirit) of the human being too.[9]

The discussion referred to is, however, not only current in the United States; there is also increasing interest in this material in the Netherlands. The openness with which religion and the meaning of life in general may again be discussed at various levels in society, has functioned as an extra stimulus to reflect on its specific place in health care. At the moment, debate in the Netherlands mainly translates into reflection on the place of *spirituality* in health care. Here, explicit talk of *religion* is largely avoided. The debate refers to what the World Health Organisation (WHO) declared in its 1998 report, namely that attention should also be paid to the spiritual aspect of heath in addition to the physical, mental and social aspects.[10] Further, the WHO in its definition of palliative care, also expressly requested that attention be paid to involving the psychological and spiritual dimensions with each other.[11]

Avoiding express talk of 'religion' might reflect the shift in the place of Christian faith in society. It occupies an equal place amidst other philosophies of life and non-Christian creeds. Multiformity and multi-culturalism presume a broader term than the concept of religion. The concept of 'spirituality' answers to this, because spirituality can be viewed as a phenomenon unifying within itself convictions, norms, values in a non-organised connection, while within religion there *is* organised connection. People who do not recognise a specific religion can also be seen as spiritual beings. However this may be: there are discussions and

---

8 Post & Vermeij, 'De gezondheidszorg als context van de geestelijke verzorging', 15-19. Medicine was practiced by priests in antiquity. When Hippocrates came on the scene, the religious and magical background to medicine was replaced as it were by his rational approach of natural philosophy. During the Middle Ages, Greco-Roman medicine survived in the Byzantine Empire. Medical knowledge was kept by monks in the monasteries. With the Enlightenment a need for empirical analysis arose, at the cost of metaphysics. Religion, or the Church, lost its authority. The split in medicine between the spiritual need of a human being and his physical suffering was a fact and would widen further as history progressed.

9 R. Toperzer, 'Considering the dangers and opportunities of pastoral care and medicine: A search for vitality, accountability and balance', in: *Journal of Health Care Chaplaincy* 7 (1998), nos 1/2, 121.

10 L.J. Tiesinga & D. Post, 'Spirituality, who cares?', in: *Verpleegkunde* (Nursing) 17 (2002) no 2, 110.

11 L.J. Tiesinga, J. Bouwer, H. Jochemsen, H. Blommestijn, K. Waaijman & D. Post, 'Spiritualiteit, (on)gezondheid en zorg: een aanwezige en onderzoekbare relatie?' (Spirituality, health and the lack of it, and care: A present, researchable relationship?), in: *Tijdschrift voor Sociale Geneeskunde* (Journal for Social Medicine) 80 (2002) no 8, 535-538.

publications on this subject in various fields.[12] Symposia are dedicated to it or are planned for the future.[13]

This collection is thus the fruit of a symposium held at the Theological University of Kampen (THUK)[14] on 24 May 2003 with the title 'Spirituality and the meaning in healthcare'. The THUK, the Stichting Geloofsovertuiging en Levensbeschouwing (SLG) (Foundation for Convictions of Faith and Philosophy of Life) and the Work group 'Research in the field of Spirituality, Health and Care' (Respire) were the co-operating agencies. Broaching this theme was an attempt to spotlight the vision of man as spiritual being and thus a seeker of meaning, promoting this as a relevant factor for a more compassionate care for both giver and seeker of care. For care is a reciprocal concept: the need of one presupposes the care of the other. That is why both 'cure' and 'care' can be unified in the concept of 'care'. This assumes that the ultimate aim of care for all the helping disciplines is in searching for the humanity of the care seeker. Everyone, from his/her own standpoint, works towards freeing the seeker of care from the evil of illness, suffering, invalidity and death. Here the dimension of spirituality is the framework of meaning for both care seeker and caregiver.

The lectures held at this symposium (most of which were given in connection with workshops), have been adapted and developed to a certain extent. The aim is a more in-depth discussion of the subject than possible during a lecture (workshop). The lectures are thematically classified into three categories. The first category contains the analysis of care practice and the fundaments of thinking on spirituality in care, the second is concerns the implementation of spirituality on the micro and meso level and the third concerns research done in this field. Two lectures are placed in every category. On more detailed substantiation, the design of this collection has the following appearance:

---

[12] See series of articles in: *Nursing* 17 (2002) no 2, 109-112; no 3, 119-123; and no 4, 220-240. See also Tiesinga et al., 'Spiritualiteit, (on)gezondheid en zorg'.

[13] On 30 November 2001 a congress took place in Amersfoort with as title 'Care for spirituality: inspired care'; on 24 May 2003 in Kampen a symposium titled 'Spirituality and meaning in health care'; and on 2 October 2003 in Amersfoort a symposium with as title 'Spirituality and health care'. On 8 October 2004 at the VUMC in Amsterdam a symposium with the working title 'Spirituality and health care' has been held. The proceedings have been published in H. Jochemsen & E. van Leeuwen, *Zinervaring in de zorg: Over de betekenis van spiritualiteit in de gezondheidszorg*, Assen: Van Gorcum, 2005. A follow-up conference is planned to be held in Zwolle in 2007.

[14] Due to a merging of the theological education of the universities of Kampen, Utrecht and Leiden on 1st January, 2007, the name of the ThUK has been changed into the Protestant Theological University.

In the category *analysis and foundation*, there are two articles concerned with the fundamentals and essence plane of care, the analysis of the context of care and the place of spirituality therein.

In the first article, *Waaijman* researches on the most profound level for the way in which spirituality manifests itself in the interaction between care seeker and caregiver. He hopes here to make a contribution to the systematic orientation of 'spirituality in care', with the study of spirituality as starting point. For the caregiver, care is profoundly relationship. This means that the competencies of the caregiver should not only float on 'the ought to be able to do' but also on an incompetent, passive component, namely that of being unable to protect oneself from the gaze of the sufferer, from being exposed to the other. Because of this exposure, the care seeker is therefore 'face' before he is anything else. According to Waaijman, without this passivity there can be no relationship, no inter-personal involvement. And without the passive space that the caregiver must be, as it were, the care seeker cannot express himself as a self-determined, independent and well-informed person. Waaijman concludes that care must understand itself as *relationship*, in its turn in various philosophy of life traditions offering access to the mercy that can be seen as the soul of care. With his contribution Waaijman not only completes the prevalent view that spirituality is a certain dimension *in* care, he advances spirituality as the *very heart* of care.

Bakker then philosophizes on the contours of the discussion on the integration of spirituality into the perception of care and the policy of care institutions. Here he focuses on the broad lines of the discussion. He analyses the present context of modern care institutions and identifies specific characteristics putting pressure on the ideal of holistic care. These are the developments around the increasing influence of technology, increase in scale, pursuit of efficiency, reduction of nursing time, transmuralisation, increasing influence of legislation, multiculturalism. The conclusion here is that these developments may cause the sick human being to be lost sight of as person, 'as unique creation of God'. Further, he also researches what the significance and relevance of the Quality Care Institutions Act (Kwaliteitswet Zorginstellingen) is to the discussion on spirituality and meaning in care – in particular article 3, in which offering spiritual care to patients who remain longer than 24 hours in a care institution is seen as a condition of qualitatively good care. This material seems to be a vague and intangible subject for managers, which leads Bakker to point out to them the importance of spiritual care when speaking of effective 'medicine'.

The second category involves the *implementation* of spirituality in care. Two levels were chosen in the context of preconditions, namely the level of the caregiver's professionalism *and* of the care institution.

In the first article *Tiesinga* inquires as to the spirituality of the nurse in particular, as a health care professional. He then familiarises himself with the call for spirituality in health care and concludes that the meaning aspect is central to it (not divisible, yet distinct from the somatic, social and psychological functioning of the human being). He subsequently concentrates on a competency profile for nurses regarding spirituality. There are also instruments allied to this, to optimise awareness around the nurses' own spiritual functioning in relationship to care. The core of the competency profile consists of the nurse being able to recognise personal values, convictions and feelings, and being able communicate about them to others. In meeting and dialoguing with the patient, the nurse is able to arrive at the co-ordination and implementation of what the patient seeks in care. To optimise his/her own competencies here, the nurse must determine on the basis of a spiritual self analysis what he/she needs to be able to give this form of care effectively. Tracing which factors play a role in the occurrence of discrepancies in the spirituality experienced between patient and professionals in care, is also something that belongs to this.

In their contribution, *Gribnau and Pijnenburg* then report on an 'integration route' which was followed within the organisation of the Radboud University Nijmegen Medical Center (UMC) from the nineties onwards, and concerned the subject of spirituality and meaning. The assumption is that in accordance with policy, this type of question is arranged in a separate service of spiritual care or pastoral service. Yet the organisation itself has also a responsibility where the great questions of direction are concerned, such as medical policy plans, policy on labour conditions and demand driven care, to mention a few issues. They defend the statement that institutions' policy agendas may and should also concern the 'soul of people, issues and institutions'. They make use of the design of quality guarantee for the description of this process: the PCDA cycle (plan, do, check and act). The UMC St Radboud from the background of its clearly described identity (Roman Catholic), has not only attempted to explicitly communicate basic assumptions, it has also tried to interpret this material on the level of education on questions of meaning (including ethics). In addition to having acknowledged both positive and less positive points of evaluation, one is more than ever aware that spirituality and meaning will be an ongoing item on the agenda and ought to be so.

In the third category, *research*, there are reports on the results of research into the role of spirituality in two contexts, namely palliative care and the supervision of cancer patients.

In the first article *Jochemsen et al.* report on empirical research that has been done into questions about life in the terminal phase of terminal patients. The aim of this research was to develop an instrument for evaluating and promoting the quality of spiritual care in terminal, palliative care, from the patient perspective. The concept of spirituality is made manageable in the research by advancing it as functional category, analogous to the model of spiritual diagnostics by George Fitchett. On the basis of data obtained from both literature research as well as semi-structured interviews with caregivers and patients concerning their needs and desires in the area of spirituality, he was able to formulate quality criteria to which spiritual care for the terminal patient must comply. These criteria are roughly ordered according to Fitchett's seven themes, but adapted to the Dutch situation. These are: faith, philosophy of life and the giving of meaning, aim in life and balance in life, experiences and emotions, courage, hope and growth, rituals and customs, relationships and social ties, and orientation and guidance. Here a distinction is made between criteria that are conditional in nature (at institutional level) and criteria that are applicable to the relationship between caregivers and patient.

Bras closes the ranks with a report on a study made into the use of meditation in the supervision of people with cancer in three centres for psycho-social supervision in the Netherlands, and of an attention training based on Vipassana meditation he himself participated in. His aim is to make a contribution to the view both on the role spirituality plays in explicitly religious forms of meditation trainings and its therapeutic significance. He begins his report with a brief summary of literature research into the significance of meditation for people with psychological and/or physical symptoms. He then describes in the light of case material the experiences gained in the Helen Dowling Institute, the Behouden Huys and the Taborhuis. To complete his research, Bras underwent an attention training (stress reduction training) in order to obtain insight into its effectiveness through participation. His conclusion is that, although no 'hard' scientific proof can be supplied on the effects of meditation, the picture demonstrated by the literature research was borne out – namely that a relaxation effect may be observed. One learns to find peace in oneself through this and to deal with the tensions around illness or pain.

This volume is concluded by an epilogue in which *Bouwer* briefly searches for common ground in the contributions offered, as well as possible points of attention that will determine the future agenda of the discussion on spirituality and meaning in health care in the Netherlands.

ANALYSIS AND FOUNDATION

K. Waaijman

SPIRITUALITY IN CARE IN THE INTERACTION BETWEEN THE PROVIDER AND SEEKER OF CARE

It is now impossible to imagine health care without spirituality. Anyone who takes the trouble to key in 'Spirituality' on medical web sites, (*Medicine, Cinahl, Invert or Picarta* for example) will encounter several hundred serious publications per annum. A few book titles at random:

Lighting the lamp. The spiritual dimension of nursing care (1994)
Spiritual competence. A model for psychiatric care (1995)
Exploring the spiritual dimension of care (1996)
Spiritual problems in nursing (1996)
Spirituality in nursing. From traditional to new age (1996)
Timeless healing. The power and biology of belief (1996)
Spiritual needs of dying patients. A methodological study (1997)
Caring from the heart. The convergence of caring and spirituality (1997)
Spirituality. The heart of nursing (1997)
The spiritual challenges of health care (1998)
Spirituality in nursing (1999)
Sacred space. Right relationship and spirituality in health care (2000)
Geloven in zorg (Believing in care) (2001)
Focus on meaning and/or religion. Nursing care in the field of spirituality (2001)
Questions on life and death in the terminal phase. Quality of spiritual care in terminal palliative care from the perspective of patients (2002)
Health care and spirituality. Listening, assessing, caring (2002)
Spirituality and intellectual disability (2002)
Psychotherapy and spirituality. Integrating the spiritual dimension into therapeutic practice (2002)
Profile of nursing competence. Care for spirituality (2002)

Anyone who quietly digests these titles will perhaps see two approaches emerge straight away. One approach sees spirituality as a specific dimension *in* care, often targeted at the competence of the care provider. The other approach perceives spirituality as the *very heart* of care. This difference in approach is not unimportant. For to the extent that emphasis is on spirituality as an aspect *within* care and to the extent this aspect is interpreted by the spiritual competence of the care provider, then to that extent the essence of the care relationship (the *very heart* of care) recedes into the background. For the character of care is not only marked by active *ability* (competence), it is equally marked by passive *sufferance*. Care is active *and* passive. And it is precisely that which makes the interaction between care provider and care seeker into a *relationship*. In turn, it is this character of relationship in care that accesses the soul of care: mercy.

A second point noticeable on further perusal of the literature, is the difference in perspectives chosen. Most publications choose the perspective of the caregiver, which usually entails the nurses. Doctors stay well out of sight. There is a lot of interest in pastoral services and in spiritual care. There is comparatively frequent discussion of spirituality in training courses. A smaller number of publications choose the perspective of the care seeker. Here, there is often a focus on serious illness (cancer, chronic illness, paralysis, dementia, aids, unbearable pain) and limited situations (palliative care, terminal care). A recurring theme is the inter-religious and intercultural reality (care for Afro-American women with diabetes; healthcare from an Islamic perspective; nursing Taiwanese woman with breast cancer; the role of the minister in Black churches, etc.)

In all this, we should consider that the literature within the field of tension between health care and spirituality reveals a richly hued prism of mentalities. Only think of alternative therapies versus the dominant mainstream course of so-called regular medical practices. In a similar manner, we see alternative spiritualities (New Age for example) versus the traditional mainstream. Some advocate healings, others view prayer as healing. Great variety in cultural and religious concepts concerning health care *and* spirituality characterize both caregivers and care seekers.

Within such a richly hued lattice of approaches, perspectives and mentalities, the methodic orientation of 'spirituality in care' is also obviously anything but simple. A jumble of strategies present itself: from abstract concepts to handy checklists; from proficiency trainings to sagacious dissertations; from all-embracing methodologies to concrete case studies. In this contribution, we whould like to add something from the discipline of spirituality studies to the methodic orientation of 'spirituality in care'. We are going to explore this orientation from two perspectives: the perspective of the caregiver and the perspective of the care seeker. In both cases, we will indicate the limitation of consciousness that is the result of a narrowing of spirituality to competence (ability, skill, active capacity). For in so doing we have quietly stripped care of its passive component, the precise thing that is fundamental to care as an event of relationship. Yet anyone who strips care of its character of relationship blocks access to the soul of care itself: mercy.

1. *The perspective of the care provider*

It would seem that from the broadening of the profile of nursing that spirituality is indeed beginning to occupy an established place within health care. Within the last few years, the factor of 'spirituality' has been added to the physical, psychological and social aspects that until recently were the only important ones in the provision of care. Thus the current *Professional profile of the nurse* assumes that the nurse, when caring for those seeking care, will allow herself to be guided by an image of humanity containing 'physical, psychological, social and spiritual aspects'.[1] The Netherlands is not alone in this. Nursing organisations abroad have also broadened their perspective with respect to the responsibility of the care provider on the issue of spiritual care: the care provider is expected to be able to name the spiritual needs of the care seeker and make, execute and evaluate an appropriate care plan.[2]

What is the tangible appearance of such a spiritual factor in care? What do those abstractly formulated ideals signify in the practice of care? I shall choose as an example the *Nursing competence profile* as developed by the Lindenboom Institute in the report *Care for spirituality*.[3] On the grounds of 28 carefully chosen studies (articles, chapters, books) six competencies were arrived at where the 'care for spirituality' was literally translated into attitudes and actions.

1. The nurse is able to maintain personal values, convictions and feelings in relationship with care seekers with different convictions about life.
2. The nurse is able to communicate his spirituality in an involved way to care seekers from different cultures.
3. The nurse is able to collect information about the spirituality of the care seeker and delineate care needs in dialogue with the care seeker.
4. In dialogue with the care seeker and in consultation with other disciplines the nurse is able to fine tune care for the care seeker's spirituality, and plan and write down a personal share in that care.
5. The nurse is able to accomplish care for the care seeker's spirituality, and evaluate that care in dialogue with the care seeker and in multi-disciplinary discussion.

---

1 E. Leistra et al., *Beroepsprofiel van de verpleegkundige* (Professional profile of the nurse), Maarssen 1999, 12.

2 See the statements of The United Kingdom Central Council for Nursing, Midwifery and Health Visiting (UKCC), The National Board for Nursing, Midwifery and Health Visiting for Scotland (NBS) and the American Association of Colleges of Nursing (AACN) in: L. Ross, 'Teaching spiritual care', in: *Nurse Education Today* 16 (1996), 38-43.

3 R. van Leeuwen & B. Cusveller, *Verpleegkundig competentieprofiel: Zorg voor spiritualiteit. Een verkennende literatuurstudie* (Nursing competence profile: Care for spirituality. An exploratory literature study), Ede 2002.

6. The nurse contributes to quality care and the advancement of professionalism in the area of care for spirituality within the care institution.

This competence profile ably assembles the most important actions and attitudes necessary to give substance to spirituality in care: the caregiver knows how to place himself regarding the spirituality of the care seeker (point 1 and 2); the caregiver is able to shape spirituality within the actual practice of nursing (point 3, 4 and 5); the caregiver makes a contribution to the quality of the care and promotes professionalism in this field (point 6). A competence profile like this can serve very well as a starting point for nursing training, where spirituality in care is taken seriously. For the profile contains a display card of skills, that could be understood as the final attainments for a training course: 'the nurse can employ… can communicate… can assemble… can co-ordinate and determine… can acomplish and evaluate… makes a contribution'.

When we list these skills, these competencies one below the other then what at first sight was hidden from our eye strikes us: the competencies are all a form of *being able*, more precisely: a form of *being able to do*. Spiritual competencies are interpreted as doable and learnable activities and attitudes. Viewed in more detail, however, there are all sorts of cracks and tears in this competence profile. For there is 'the relationship with the care seekers', with whom there is communication 'in a concerned way', with whom there is 'dialogue'. But anyone who talks about relationship, involvement and dialogue, introduces categories that cannot be contained in terms of doable actions and attitudes. Something continues to adhere to these categories that cannot be planned and for which, in the strictest sense, no one is 'competent', in that we are continually surprised by it. That the other person gazes at us, moves us through his need – this is what we cannot defend ourselves against. We are passive on this point and to a certain extent 'incompetent'. We give in. We cannot bear it. Here we submit, endure, are passive. Anyone who rereads the 28 studies analysed by the Lindenboom Institute from this perspective, will have little trouble in discovering this passive dimension over and over again; it is, however, given no thematic place in the competence profile of the caregiver. Wrongly so, for although this dialogic *in*-competence is not learnable and doable, one can be *aware* of it. And that is precisely a question of spirituality for the caregiver, but also as we shall see, for the care seeker.

To obtain a sharper image of what I mean by this *incompetence*, I will briefly describe what I learned during the course 'Meaning in Care', given on seven wards of the University Medical Centre St Radboud in Nijmegen. Around 150 students participated in this course, based on the experiences of nurses (doctors were rather conspicuous by their absence). The point of departure was always:

what touches you in your work? What inspires you? What can't you shower off in the evening when you get home? There were two clearly differentiated components in the caregivers' answers: an active and a passive one.

The active component expressed itself in words such as: 'help', 'matter to the patient', 'show that you are there', 'hold a hand for a little while'. They wish to listen well, listen to the story behind the story of the one asking for help, etc. Here the one offering help is practicing her profession (vocation is avoided). Words are uttered like: professionalism and quality improvement. Collegiality is of essential importance in this work. All together this characterizes the active component in the care relationship: you can do it, you can learn it, you can dedicate yourself to it, you can work on it together. This active component is explicitly propounded in roughly fifty statements. One caregiver says: 'The work makes you what you are. You are a great deal. You go through a lot, which makes you realize who you are and what you are doing'.

The passive component is less public than the active one. It leads a secret life, in the shadow of professional identity. There is little room for it institutionally. It is privatized. This passive component was expressed in roughly 100 statements in words such as: 'having to look on patiently', 'bumping against limitations', 'facing questions to which you do not know the answer', 'moved by suffering', 'having to look at death in the eye', 'exposed to feelings of fear and indignation, powerlessness and insecurity'. 'Oh, isn't not being able to do anything difficult,' sighed one caregiver. Main factors in the passive component of the caregiver are the following.

1. The nurse knocks against the personal world of the care seeker, who has his or her own stubborn opinions about the illness and recovery process, who falls back on basic needs, who wants to live at whatever cost or alternatively wants to die as quickly as possible, who searches for certainties that are not there, who effortlessly blames his illness on God or is absolutely counting on Him to cure him, who invariably hauls a whole family into the hospital or alternatively is all alone. The caregiver must patiently look on, is passive.
2. Care is risky. There are many advisors, but when care fails there is only one responsible: the caregiver. Feelings of powerlessness and insecurity are released: 'I get really fed up with my powerlessness'. When something has almost but not quite gone wrong: 'I'm still shaking when I lie in bed that evening'.
3. Suffering deeply moves the caregiver: 'When you see someone suffering, then that moves you'. Especially when this suffering is accompanied by loss of identity, mutilation, humiliation, and of course death. 'We see many people who are seriously ill, but when they really get to hear that things

look very bad, that affects me deeply. Then you think. Oh my God, what am I going to do?' Especially when the caregiver has been with the patient now entering into the terminal phase for a long time: 'I quite often cry for patients'.

4. Emotional intensity is reinforced when the nurse identifies with the patient; this repeatedly occurs in spite of prior warning. Who is so hardened that he cannot be moved if someone of similar age, a colleague, or a small child is involved? 'What saddens me the most is when I see someone come in with a child. Then my eyes can fill with tears at the sight of that parent. I can't bear to think that something like that might happen to my child. When that happens, I just don't understand anything anymore'.

Why is this passive component in care so important? Because this passive component is essential for the care relationship. Martin Buber, the Jewish philosopher who spent his whole life pondering relationship, encounter, connections and reciprocity states unequivocally: 'I become the "Thou", becoming, I say Thou'.[4] That is to say: you touch me, appeal to me. I can not organize that in any way at all. I am passive: I am touched by him. My only real answer to this passive contact is that I say yes to it. Only then do I *really* respect the other person. I-becoming-to-the-Thou that I meet, *that* is my answer to my Thou. Relationship between people arises precisely there where I am touched by a Thou and where I say yes to this touch. Emmanuel Levinas, another Jewish philosopher who has developed this dialogic thinking, emphasises time and time again passivity with respect to the other as a core moment in the relationship. This concerns a divine weakness in man, existing in the impossibility of remaining indifferent towards another's need: 'I can not withdraw from the countenance of a fellow human being without failing and without making a slip or without getting a complex'.[5] The humanity of the human being is damaged if I do not endorse my passivity with respect to the other. Levinas calls this an 'impossible indifference – towards the misery and the lapses of the other, the imperative responsibility with respect to him'.[6] The other in his need disturbs me, addresses me, cannot be evaded: 'Ceaseless agitation of anxiety, utmost passivity in the responsibility for the responsibility of the other'.[7] Levinas does not tire of pointing out the essence of humanity in this 'response-ability' (*responsibilité*) with respect to the other: 'Putting subjectivity in this responsibility is: to note a passivity that is never passive enough through being digested by the other'.[8]

---

4 M. Buber, *Ich und Du* (I and Thou), Köln 1966, 18.

5 E. Levinas, *De Dieu qui vient à l'idée* (The God who comes to the Idea), Paris 1982, 118.

6 Ibid., 116.

7 Ibid., 120.

8 Ibid., 119.

Now back to the care situation. We saw how good it is that the spiritual dimension in care is gaining shape, in addition to the physical, psychological and social aspects. We also saw how this spiritual aspect may be actualized in a competence profile: communicating with the care seeker in a concerned way that proceeds from his culture and philosophy of life. Charting the spirituality of the care seeker and gearing care to it, improving quality care in this manner. But above all, we saw that the factor 'active-*capability*' dominates so powerfully in this competence profile that in-competence is being pushed aside. We have just seen that it is precisely this 'passivity/inability', 'weakness', 'anxiety', 'becoming-the-Thou' that partly creates the relationship. Indeed this is noted in the literature of care, time after time. Steemers-Van Winkoop in *Geloven in Zorg* (Faith in Care) thus poses that relationship is *the* precondition for acknowledging and working with the spirituality of the sick person.[9] And, in turn, a relationship assumes that the nurse feels how she is moved, how her own experience changes through the patient's situation.

Conclusion: care is relationship at its most profound. Without relationship, no care. But relationship implies passivity, baring oneself to the other. Without passivity, no relationship: I become through my relationship to the Thou, as I become I say Thou. The care competence can flourish on the humus layer of the care relationship. But if active, self determining, doable, learned competence – even if it concerns the spiritual dimension of the care seeker! – dominates, then it blocks the essentially passive care relationship and with it the very soul of care: mercy.

2. *The perspective of the care seeker*

Recent decades have demonstrated an important shift in the perspective of the care seeker. This perspective has been traditionally determined by the insights of the well-meaning doctor. It was termed the paternalistic type. Strong and weak forms of paternalism are discernable here. In strong paternalism one takes action and interferes in the patient's life, if he is acting in conflict with his long-term chances for life. It makes no difference here whether he is in full possession of his faculties and is acting after careful deliberation, or whether he is physically or mentally disturbed. Weak paternalism merely applies restrictions to liberty in the latter case.[10]

---

9 M. Steemers-Van Winkoop, *Geloven in zorg: Omgaan met geloof, levensbeschouwing en spiritualiteit in de gezondheidszorg* (Faith in care), Baarn 2001.

10 D. Birnbacher, 'Selbstmord und Selbstmortbehütung' (Suicide and suicide prevention), in: A. Leist (Ed.), *Um Leben und Tod* (About life and death), Frankfurt a.M. 1990, 395-422.

In recent decades, the perspective of patient autonomy has challenged medical paternalism. Key words are: right to self-determination, independence, patient centred and demand-driven care, right of decision, right of information. In short: respect for the autonomy of the care seeker. 'The principle of patient autonomy has shifted the doctor-patient relationship from dependence on the doctor to participation in decision making. The patient may well be fearful, vulnerable and dependent due to his illness, but this weakness does not take the moral right away from him to affect the decisions that concern him'.[11] Not much imagination is necessary to see that the autonomy of the care seeker is a perfect mirror image of the competence of the care provider. In both cases an appeal is made to the skill of an emancipated self.

What does the 'competent' spirituality of the autonomous care seeker look like? Three aspects of the spirituality of the care seeker may be distinguished.[12]

1. *Everyday spirituality*. The care seeker imparts information about the spirituality known to him from his ordinary, everyday life and which he wishes to see continued. This everyday spirituality – seen from the perspective of the care seeker! – may contain all sorts of elements: his philosophy of life as background, main outlines of his life story, the meaning of spiritual experiences, certain spiritual practices and symbols. This ordinary spirituality may be important to the care seeker in living through the illness and healing process. Moreover, prayer, meditation, reading certain texts and participation in gatherings may have consequences for care provision.
2. *The spirituality of being ill*. When someone is confronted with illness, then everyday spirituality kicks in. The consequences are unpredictable. For some, deeper layers in their everyday spirituality are tapped, while for others everyday spirituality is (for a while) pushed into the background or seems unreliable. Some are led to acceptance or to realistic appraisal by their everyday spirituality, while for others an in itself vigorous everyday spirituality turns into rebellion or depression. Illness may cast the

[11] E. Pellegrino, 'Die medische Ethik in den USA: Die Situation heute und die Aussichten für Morgen (Medical Ethics in the USA: The situation today and the prospects for tomorrow), in: H. Sass (Ed.), *Bioethik in den USA: Methoden, Themen, Positionen* (Bioethics in the USA: Methods, themes, positions), Berlin-Heidelberg-New York 1988, 1-20.

[12] See for this J. de Wolf, 'Verpleegkundige beroepsverantwoordelijkheid in samenwerkingsrelaties' (Professional responsibility for nurses in co-operative relationships), in: B. Cusveller (Ed.), *Volwaardige verpleging: Morele beroepsverantwoordelijkheid in de zorgverlening* (Complete nursing. Moral professional responsibility in care), Amsterdam 1999; R. van Leeuwen & B. Cusveller, *Verpleegkundig competentieprofiel: Zorg voor spiritualiteit*, Ede 2002, 8.

care seeker into spiritual affliction because everyday spirituality cannot place elements such as crisis, wretchedness or powerlessness.[13]

3. *Imbalanced spirituality.* No single spirituality is completely in balance, for then it is dead. But sometimes a spirituality is thrown greatly off balance: an excess of asceticism, neurotic practice of prayer, delusions or compulsive images, extreme fear of God's punitive hand, etc. Sometimes a lopsided spiritual growth is one of the causes of the illness, or spiritual derailment influences care giving in a negative way.

It is part of the care seeker's autonomy and his presumed competence (ideally) to convey information on his spirituality in any way to the care provider. But as I write this, doubts and questions spring to mind: How is it possible to talk about your everyday spirituality in times of crisis? Is not this spirituality now out of balance *per se*? Is there not a lot of time necessary before a crisis can demonstrate its curative power? And sometimes there seems to be nothing curative about it at all! Is not much power of discernment necessary to give the correct information? In borderline cases, are we not completely delivered unto a well-meaning ear? Care seeker autonomy has accordingly (just like the caregiver competence) its limits and its downside too – its *in*-competence.

We would like to explore this downside further in the light of the study by Christoph Holzems, *Patient Autonomy*.[14] The thinking behind patient autonomy has been followed as far as possible in this study, and from different perspectives. Yet the author keeps on knocking against the limits of a fully considered care seeker autonomy. The limits of this autonomy ideal become visible precisely where the care seeker reaches his limits: becomes completely confused (dementia), can no longer express himself (coma), is at the end of his strength (euthanasia), no longer desires medical information, etc. It is precisely in these borderline situations that the autonomy of the care seeker is shown to be an empty ideal and he is easy prey for a revitalised paternalism. 'For a paternalistic medical practice would connect to verbal championing of patient autonomy in this way: it would only be necessary to demonstrate that the ideal patient would assent to a certain therapy, for one to view oneself as authorized to judge this therapy applicable to this actual patient with his restricted decision

[13] For the richly hued gamut of reactions of ordinary spirituality in the case of sickness see K. Waaijman, *Psalmen bij ziekte en genezing* (Psalms for sickness and healing), Kampen 1981. See also the four special issues of *Speling* 32 (1980) which are about sickness and spirituality.

[14] C. Holzem, *Patientenautonomie: Bioethische Erkundungen über einen funktionalen Begriff der Autonomie im medizinischen Kontext* (Patient autonom, bioethical: About a functional concept of autonomy in medical context), Münster-Hamburg-London 1998.

competence'.[15] It is not, however, necessary at all to be critically ill to knock against the limits of his competence. 'Many medical decisions are so difficult (especially when diagnosis or prognosis is uncertain and a complex grid of probable factors has to be considered) that they would demand too much of the patient even in times of health, let alone when he is conditioned by the agitation, fear and depression that accompany illness'.[16]

Christoph Holzem, confronted with the actual limits of the care seeker competence, rightly states that the care relationship as the actual fundament of patient autonomy should undergo rethinking. 'For both human experience and philosophical reflection show that real autonomy is possible through successful "with-each-other" and in the recognition of the other as the other. Autonomy is therefore essentially a discursive, dialogic event'.[17] Within the dialogue between caregiver and care seeker the care seeker may convey what he has to say as best he can (independence). But much more importantly, the care seeker can utter in the dialogue what *cannot* be expressed in words, but is wordlessly communicated at the same time: 'I am so vulnerable. Do not strip me. Do not let me die'. This wordless statement precedes all information, competence and autonomy. This wordless statement creates the care relationship:

> Structures of relationship within the world of medicine are essentially characterized by the anthropological paradigms of need and help, in particular however by the vulnerability of the sick patient. Illness changes the examination of self in the first place, as well as observation of the world and of the personal future. Illness is an ontological attack on the person and on the life of the individual patient.[18]

In his illness, the sick person shares his vulnerability and his need for help. Without using competent words he has already frankly expressed his incompetence. And that incompetence is still more reinforced by the necessity of exposing himself further: 'The vulnerability we experience as a result of our illness is increased by the fact that we must expose our body, our personal life and our personal history in order to admit the possibility of benefaction. We have to entrust the things we are most deeply concerned about to the health

[15] L. Kuttig, 'Autonomie zwischen ethischen Anspruch und medizinischer Wirklichkeit (Autonomy between ethical responsibility and medical reality), in: L. Eckersberger & U. Gähde (Eds.), *Ethische Norm und empirische Hypothese* (Ethical norm and empirical hypothesis), Frankfurt a.M. 1993, 279-280; also see O. O'Neil, 'Paternalism and partical autonomy', in: *Journal of Medical Ethics* 10 (1984), 174-175.

[16] D. Birnbacher, 'Patientenautonomie und ärztliche Ethik am Beispiel der prädiktiven Diagnostik' (Patient autonomy and medical ethics in examples of predictive diagnostics), in: *Jahrbuch für Wissenschaft und Ethik* (Annual for Science and Ethics) 2 (1997), 110.

[17] Holzem, *Patientenautonomie*, 17; also see 216-217, 329-336, 372-374.

[18] Ibid., 350.

experts'.[19] In his illness the sick person reveals his fundamental vulnerability and need of help. This statement of self is listened to in the care relationship so that revealing oneself further is not experienced as injurious. The care seeker conveys this *prior to* all further information. Female participants within the medical debate had already responded to this 'other voice' in the Eighties, particularly Carol Gilligan.[20]

The other voice of the one asking for help can sometimes be at odds with his competence. I have to think of the story of someone infected with the HIV virus eighteen years ago.[21] He works in health care where he encounters seriously disheartened people almost on a daily basis. His internist is 'a serious man, but not without humour', who has become very important to him, both as a doctor and a human being.

> We fight a silent battle over the seriousness of my situation and how to deal with it. I think that he finds me too laconic when, medically speaking, something is difficult or wrong again. I can well understand his worry; I'm often worried too. Yet I keep seeing the sun. I play down unpleasant messages. I inflate good news. I am duly aware of that. By doing this I see a chance of reining in discouragement and fear and strengthening expectation and hope.[22]

We see here a seriously ill person, who himself works in health care, who acts with the same lack of reflection as a healthy person: He is saying something concerning discouragement and expectation, fear and hope, beyond all 'seriousness' and 'worry'. Beaten back to the remaining 'here and now', a 'wonderful buoyancy' arises that breaches the 'seriousness' of the competent conversation between doctor and patient.

> Sometimes this attitude is misunderstood; I'm bothered by that, especially if professionals do it. Hope is encased in the buoyancy: not wishing-in-spite-of-knowing-better to become better, but a matured desire to live the good life as long as possible and to experience life as good. To recognize this human condition, professionals will have to dare to confront their own vulnerability and fear. Then they can stand by the seriously ill patient.[23]

This is said by a care seeker who is himself a caregiver!

---

[19] V. Sharp, 'Justice and care: The implications of the Kohlberg-Gilligan debate for medical ethics', in: *Theoretical Medicine* 13 (1992), 308.

[20] C. Gilligan, *In a different voice: Psychological theory and women's development*, Cambridge-London 1982. For a brief overview, see Holzem, *Patientenautonomie*, 337-341.

[21] C.S., 'Leven met een ernstige onvoorspelbare ziekte: Een persoonlijke ervaring' (Life with a serious, unpredictable illness: a personal experience), in: V. Kirkels & H. Rouwenhorst (Eds.), *Hoop als helpende hand: Een medische verkenning met filosofische en pastorale kanttekeningen* (Hope as helping hand: A medical investigation with philosophical and pastoral notes), Nijmegen 2003, 23-29.

[22] Ibid., 28-29.

[23] Ibid., 29.

We began with the autonomy of the seeker of help: his independence, his competent self-determination. This is very important in care, certainly for verbal and non verbal communication on the issue of spirituality. But beyond every communication something wordless is communicated: 'I am so vulnerable. Do not strip me. Do not let me die'. This wordless statement of self with which the care seeker entrusts himself to the other, creates the care relationship. The philosopher Emmanuel Levinas previously referred to, calls this statement of self: the face. Face means: be-ing in nakedness. One usually covers this face with 'whats' (information, competencies, self-determination, autonomy). One asks after content, after nouns, after adjectives. What do you do? What do you want? What do you think of it? But the person who must answer these questions 'has already *presented himself* without being a "content". He has presented himself as a face [...] To the question *who?* Answers the non-qualifiable presence of an existent who presents *himself* without reference to anything'.[24] Face is: 'the being naked of being' of someone opposite me. Where someone exposes himself, he is face. Therefore the whole body can express being face, even 'a hand or a curving of the shoulder'.[25]

Conclusion: when the care relationship is really relationship, then the care seeker is above all face: do not let me die. He exposes himself to the gaze of the other. This exposure is rather incompetent than competent self-determination, rather surrender than autonomy, rather wordless presence than independence. The face of the care seeker immediately appeals to the caregiver with the inescapable authority of the weak. Within this appeal, the self-determined, independent and well-informed care seeker can express himself. But if this independent competence becomes dominant in well-meant patient autonomy – even if the patient gives us maximum information about his spirituality – then this competence will still block a more essential incompetence, which creates the care relationship.

3. Care relationship

We have looked at care from two perspectives: that of the caregiver and that of the care seeker. Both perspectives are understood as active components within the modern culture of care: the caregiver gives a profile of his professional competence, the care seeker deploys his independent self-determination. Applied to spirituality in care this means: The person providing aid develops his competence

[24] E. Levinas, *Totality and Infinity: An essay on exteriority* (trans. A. Lingis), Pittsburgh (PA) 2000 (14th print), 177 (Orig. publ. 1961).

[25] Ibid., 240.

profile on the point of spirituality in care; the person asking for aid articulates his everyday spirituality and attempts to say what the illness has done with that spirituality.

We also saw, however, that the passive dimension in the caregiver and care seeker is obscured through this one sided emphasis on the active aspects: the caregiver is touched, affected, moved by the sick person: the care seeker requests above all: 'Do not let me die'. This 'other voice' is difficult to hear and is easily silenced. That is why we have paid so much attention to it.

The caregiver *and* the care seeker are both active *and* passive at the same time. It is precisely that which makes a care relationship. It is precisely where the caregiver is touched in his soul by the sick person, that the relationship comes into being: 'I become the "Thou"; as becoming say I you'. It is precisely where the care seeker wordlessly says: 'Help me!', that he bears himself, exposes his countenance, makes himself present. Within this care relationship, the caregiver and the care seeker can now unfold their mutual competence, even on the point of spirituality – without becoming inhuman. Essential, however, to this competence-spirituality is the relationship-spirituality preceding it. The care relationship is essential to care spirituality.

This relationship character of care, anchored in mutual passivity and incompetence, is splendidly expressed in the double origin of the word 'care'. For there are two ways of explaining our word 'care'.[26] The first possibility assumes the Old Indian *surksati*, which means: he is concerned about somebody. This basic meaning resounds in nuances of meaning such as: take care of (taking the trouble to keep someone alive, exert oneself for someone, dedicate yourself to his welfare) assume care for something (know responsibility, deem oneself committed). The active line primarily expresses itself in this etymology: dedicate oneself actively and competently to someone's life and welfare, from an attitude of involvement and responsibility. It would be incorrect to unilaterally endow the care provider with this active significance. The care seeker has also, as we saw, his own competence: to take on the responsibility for the sickness and cure process.

But there is another explanation of the word 'care'. This is based on the original form *sorgo*, to be found in several languages.[27] This second origin resounds in nuances of meaning such as: have a care (danger, difficulties, threat to life), sunk in cares (feelings of fear and worry) that which arouses care, makes me care and takes care that I have grey hair and sleepless nights. The passive line in

---

[26] Zie J. Franck & N. van Wijk, *Franck's etymologisch woordenboek* (Etymological dictionary), 's-Gravenhage 1949^2, 827 en 870; P.A.F. van Veen, *Etymologisch woordenboek*, Utrecht-Antwerpen 1989, 839; *Het Woordenboek der Nederlandsche Taal*, Utrecht 1996, 2255.

[27] Compare the Irish *serg*, the Lithuanian *sergu*, the old church slavic *sragu*.

care primarily emerges in this second etymology: passive and incompetent are subject to that which arouses cares, that gives me cares. It would be incorrect to delegate this passive side of care to the care seeker alone. The caregiver is sunk in cares from time to time too, simply because the cares of the sick person touch him. This passive dimension of care takes care, as we have seen, that there is an element of human relationship in care.

We also find both lines of significance in the Anglo-Saxon duo *care/cure*. These two words both go back to the Latin word *curare*. Four nuances of meaning are differentiated here.[28]

1. Via the Germanic *cara*, meaning 'problem' or 'sadness', we come to the field of significance of fear, pain, misery, grief and psychological suffering.
2. A fundamental attitude of care towards people and institutions: feeling that something is significant and valuable and that people care about it.
3. A practical attitude, expressing concern about someone, as against a formal attitude, expressing distance to them in a chilly, business-like fashion; a empathetic attitude that is personally involved.
4. An attitude to life arising from and fed by inter-personal involvement. We clearly see the passive component (sadness, fear, suffering) *and* the active component (consideration, solicitude) playing a role in these four nuances of meaning. Furthermore both components are included in interpersonal involvement. Warren Reich thus correctly states:

> Care is a contemporary concept that is related to friendship and love, but has a distinctive characteristic of its own, particularly in the medical setting. It is a virtue whereby one person is inclined to pay close and respectful attention to the other and to offer service to the other in a relationship that is characterized by commitment to help the other grow, in part by helping the other care for him/herself, so that the one being cared for (the one for whom one shows compassion) is not simply a recipient of services but one who thereby is enabled to care for self and others.[29]

We see the active *and* the passive component afresh: the person who *is* cared for, is at the same time someone who is enabled to *care* for himself and for the other person. Both moments are emphatically expressed as 'relationship', characterized by mutual involvement.

It is of essential importance for the orientation of 'spirituality in care' to keep an eye on this relational connection. The active-passive structure of action and

[28] Cf. W. Reich, 'The history of the notion of care', in: idem (Ed.), *Encyclopedia of Bioethics*, New York 1995^2, 319-331.

[29] W. Reich, 'Models of pain and suffering: Foundations for an ethic of compassion', in: *Acta Neurochirurgica Supplement* 38 (1987), 118.

the interpersonal involvement interlock immediately. A core sentence from *Ich und Du* by Martin Buber is: 'The Thou meets me. But I step into direct relationship with it. Hence the relation means being chosen and choosing, suffering and action in one'.[30] I am passive/suffering because the Thou encounters me, touches me (I come to the Thou). But this passivity/sufferance (my emotion) asks to be actively involved in the Thou: I becoming (to the Thou) say I Thou. It means growth in relationship, when 'my action (my choice for Thou) increasingly 'resembles my suffering' (my being chosen by Thou).[31]

Conclusion: it is essential for care to understand itself as *relationship,* as interpersonal involvement. The necessary condition for that, however, is that not only the active component in the care relationship should be developed (competency, autonomy), but equally that attention should be paid to the passive component (emotion, vulnerability). For it is the passive component that gives rise to the care relationship (I become to Thou), in order to be completed by the active component (I becoming I say Thou).

4. *Mercy, the soul of care*

Why dwell so long on care as a relationship, established as a passive-active structure of action? Why dwell so long on care itself, while we speak of spirituality of/in care? There are two reasons for this.

The first reason arises from the specific place that care (just like education, management, mass media, etc.) takes up within the entirety of spirituality. Spirituality of/in care is no school of spirituality (such as for instance the order of Benedictines or a Sufi monastery). It is a 'secular' form of spirituality, rooted in laicism, in which the course of a life, birth, upbringing, residence and work, mutual involvement and care are central data of immediate importance for the spirituality that is experienced.[32] Well, what applies to all spiritualities applies very particularly to the laic spiritualities: 'The essence of every spirituality is not an elsewhere outside the language of time. It is the language of time taken seriously by the spiritual person'.[33] Applied to care: we should not try to implant a spirituality from outside. We should listen to the language of care itself. That is the first reason why we – for the sake of spirituality! – should listen so carefully

30 M. Buber, *Ich und Du* (I and Thou), Köln 1966, 18.

31 Ibidem.

32 See for a description of this laical spirituality in secular contexts K. Waaijman, *Spirituality: Forms, foundations, methods*, Leuven etc. 2002, 18-115.

33 M. De Certeau, 'Cultures et spiritualités' (Cultures and spirituality)', in: *Concilium* 2 (1966) no 9, 11.

to care itself. What is care? How do the active and passive components relate to each other? What does the relationship profile of care look like? These are all direct questions of spirituality. They are prior to inquiry into the spiritual aspects (in addition to the physical, social and psychological aspects) that must be built into care as an improvement of the competency profile of the care seeker. Care itself is the form and location of care spirituality.

The second reason is directly connected to this. If care is not understood as an active-passive involvement event, then we cut it off from its being, from the source that inspires it: mercy. For whatever term used to denote mercy–benevolence, compassion, mercy, pity, commiseration, clemency, selfless aid, or whatever –, it is always about a duality of emotion and help, being moved and effort, passivity and activity. Well, it is obvious that care is cut off from mercy when one robs it of its active-passive involvement structure. That is the reason for the ongoing emphasis on the passive component in care, in addition to its active component. That is also why the relationship aspect of care is emphasised. For the two together give access to mercy, which is the actual spiritual seat of care. The importance of this spiritual seat is not only underlined from the point of view of spirituality or the Christian tradition. The medical world itself increasingly views compassion as one of the most essential aspects of care:

> the sympathy with, the com-passio, is a reaction to the suffering of the patient and emerges within this context as the virtue of the doctor. [...] It is particularly in contemporary everyday practice of medicine that there are complaints of a lack of mercy and, above all, of compassion. This virtue will not be captured in principles, rules, directives or a catalogue of duties. Compassion is a habitual disposition of this person. It has to be recognized here that compassion may only be experienced from the perspective of the sufferer.[34]

Within the medical world itself, mercy appears as an essential basic component of care.[35]

Where care retains its active-passive structure of action and, along with this, its relationship character, it is an entry to the spiritual region of mercy, which is a central fact in all great spiritualities.

1. *Biblical spirituality*. In bible spirituality this mercy is expressed by two concepts: the active movement of granting (*chesed*) and the passive movement of tenderness (*rechamim*). The impulse to grant wells up spontaneously in the heart and flows abundantly. It focuses on the other, wishing to oblige the other. It works carefully and inventively. It leaves the other be. While it

[34] Holzem, *Patientenautonomie*, 352 and 354.

[35] Ibid., 351, 351, 357.

gives itself away in love, it knows that everything depends on its reception by the beneficiary. Tenderness is: being touched to the heart by the sight of the other person, which releases in me a flow that knows no bounds. Yet it does not carry me away, for I can choose to lend myself to its dynamic or not. Tenderness seeks to crystallise itself in tender expressions: reconciliation, care, caressing. Grace and tenderness often go together (Zech 7:9; Jer 16:5; Hos 2:21; Dan 1:9; Isa 63:7; Ps 25:6; 40:12; 51:3; 69:17; 103:4; 106:45-46; Lam 3:22.). This in no way signifies that they are synonymous. On the contrary, their dynamic is different: the impulse to grant springs from the spontaneous desire to do good, tenderness is aroused by the other; granting shows itself in the a sovereign will that transports the giving from within, tenderness is released, it is also a weakness that glitters, it cannot contain itself. There are also similarities. Both are characterized by abundance: in granting, giving is abundant as a blossoming tree in spring, tenderness breaches the dikes. Both are characterized by seeking actualisation: granting goes to work in a craftsman-like, careful and inventive way, tenderness leavens all its works with tender softness. Both are marked by reciprocity: granting waits until the other can receive that which is given, tenderness allows itself to be carried along in the joy of reconciliation.[36]

2. *Jewish spirituality*. Mercy is central to Jewish spirituality. The term 'chassidisme' – derived from chesed, meaning mercy in effect – was repeatedly the key word for spirituality and mysticism. God's abundant goodness is central to all Chassidic spiritualities. Chassidim rejoice in the grace of God and attempt to receive this in their life and to express it. All areas of life are involved in this, not just the specifically religious. The everyday ones such as eating, drinking, sleeping, working, dancing, desires, strange thoughts, etc are involved too.
3. *Christian spirituality*. Jesus was a teacher of mercy: 'your loyalty to the Law must surpass' (Mt 5:20), 'your left hand must not know what your right hand is doing' (Mt 5:3; 6:3-4), 'I tell you not to resist evil' (Mt 5:39), 'go two miles if anyone asks you to go one mile' (Mt 5:41), 'love your enemies' (Mt 5:44), 'do not judge others' (Mt 7:1), etc. The beatitudes summarise this mentality in one sentence: 'Oh the bliss of those whose strength is in their gentleness, for they shall enter into possession of the earth' (Mt 5:7). We see the same image in Luke, especially in the parable of the merciful father that 'he was heart-sorry for him' (Lk 15:20) embraces his lost son, and the parable of the Good Samaritan who 'was heart-sorry when

[36] For a more detailed description of mercy in the Scriptures, see K. Waaijman, 'Gunst en vertedering: Barmhartigheid in het Oude Testament' (Grace and tenderness: Mercy in the Old Testament), in: *Speling* 51 (1999) no 1, 52-59.

he saw the state he was in' (Lk 10:33) cares for a badly wounded traveller. Luke's sermon turns on this one sentence: 'You must show yourself merciful as your Father is merciful' (Lk 6:36).

4. *Islamic spirituality*. Almost all chapters in the Koran begin with the opening sentence: 'In the name of God, the Merciful one, the Compassionate one…'. The devout Moslem in following God strives to make God's mercifulness his own by humaneness, friendliness, helpfulness, compassion and selfless love. Hereby the devout person continually repeats the name of God as 'Compassionate One', in doing so being able to experience his own deeds of mercy as deeds of God: they are stripped inwardly of selfishness, the need for applause, the desire for reward and appreciation.
5. *Buddhist spirituality*. Compassion (*karuna*) is a form of love that does not stem from the I, but from the other. Pity is cultivated together with friendliness, empathetic joy and equanimity. Friendliness delivers happiness to the other person, an empathetic joy is happy with the other's happiness; equanimity frees a person from attachment to the attitudes just named. This creates opportunity for compassion: emotion for the other emanating from the other. A well-known sutra from the *Pali* canon says: 'As a mother protects her own son, her only child with her life, so should we unfold our spirit to all living beings. Unfold the spirit without limit, full of compassion for the whole world' (*Metta sutra*). This compassion manifests itself in deeds: giving alms, assisting people in need, being good to animals, being thankful, giving food to the poor and food, digging wells alongside a main road, etc.
6. *Taoist spirituality*. Everything revolves around *tao*: the Motion that bears everything like a primitive mother and infuses all things. We come into contact with this silent Source by acting without premeditation, called *wu-wei*, a quiet equanimity that does not interfere, but allows the Motion to take its course. Non-doing yields to the Fundamental Motion of man and objects, bringing them back to their original Emotion. Coming to this gentle sympathetic movement is a way of purification: distortions, constraints and contortions are released. The Way fulfils its movement in utter stillness; silent attention guards its being.

Conclusion: Mercy, a central fact in every spirituality, is the spiritual region of care – concern for another's need. For mystics, each care situation is an invitation to practice mercy in the footsteps of the merciful Compassionate One. 'Be merciful as your heavenly Father is merciful'. Every care situation is an invitation to receive Divine Compassion and to go inward to what we must thank our existence to and on which our ultimate salvation depends. Care gives access to divine Mercy and flows forth from it.

D.J. Bakker

SPIRITUALITY AND MEANING IN HEALTH CARE PERCEPTION AND POLICY

Introduction

In article 3 of the Care Institutions (Quality) Act[1] legislation instructs the care provider to offer spiritual care to patients staying in institutions of care for at least 24 hours. This is to be co-ordinated with the religious convictions of the patients or clients as far as possible.

The evaluation of this Act carried out in 2001 demonstrated that concerted action between the various bodies responsible is still too informal. Tasks and responsibilities have still not come into their own sufficiently. The Act assumes the systematics of conditioned self-regulation, decentralising responsibility to those operating in the field.

Attention to spirituality and meaning making are often considered synonymous with spiritual care. Spirituality and meaning therefore often come up for discussion as such, in institutions' perceptions of health care. On the one hand, it has to be said that management in care institutions – administration, board of directors – often has great trouble giving content and a place in policy to such things. To managers they are vague concepts. A more workable definition of spirituality and meaning should be developed that management can also apply. On the other hand, the question arises whether care institutions do actually have the time and the space to pay attention to questions of spirituality and meaning in our times, certainly with respect to hospitals which are naturally focused on as rapid a diagnosis and therapy as possible.

The 24-hour criterion is mentioned in the Quality Act. It concerns patients who stay in care institutions for at least 24 hours. This is occurring less and less frequently. Complicated and intrusive treatments may be carried out in outpatient clinics to an increasing degree. Do these patients also have need of

---

[1] Kwaliteitswet Zorginstellingen (KZI) 1996. (Care Institutions Quality Act)

spiritual care? We researched this within the Academic Medical Centre in Amsterdam and published the results in the report 'Short Day'.[2]

In addition to the above mentioned increase in outpatient treatment, there are a number of developments in modern hospitals making attention to spirituality and meaning quite difficult. We will briefly discuss them at a later point in this contribution.

Another complication is the fact that when spirituality and meaning are part of the care given, the tie-up to it outside the hospital is often completely lacking, due to increasing individualisation and secularisation. 'Transmural' (the co-ordination of intramural and extramural care) care projects and pathways demonstrate this. It is often much more difficult to transfer the patient 'spiritually' to extramural assistance than it is to do so 'medically'. People no longer have links to Churches, and social networks are also increasingly lacking. Domicilliary care has long waiting lists and the care given has to be accounted for in minutes. Care provision in the family context, volunteer assistance, is often absent in urban environments in the West of the country. Volunteer organisations do good work but naturally cannot do everything.

An interesting question for management is 'how many partialities in the ideological sphere' should be made available in the institution, and who will pay for this. Should these people be employed by the hospital or can we 'outsource' this to an institution that trains spiritual carers and 'hires' them out to care institutions?

Health insurance companies are very unresponsive where any separate financing of this sort of care is concerned, and are usually of the opinion that it 'should all be in the budget' (the same goes for the Ministry of Health for that matter). Giving substance to and organising some matters is too often dependent on the personal slant and preference of management.

There are a great many different care institutions in the Netherlands. They include large and small hospitals, nursing and care homes, institutions caring for the mental and physically handicapped, etc. Naturally, questions concerning spirituality and meaning will be posed differently in different institutions and the answers will be different. Questions and problems mentioned will be introduced and discussed in more detail in this article.

In this contribution our starting point is the large general (academic) hospital.[3]

---

2 J.E. de Vries & M. van Gilst, *Kort dag: Rapportage van de peiling Poliklinische Geestelijke Verzorging in het AMC*, Amsterdam 2001.

3 D.J. Bakker, 'Het algemene ziekenhuis van onze tijd: Pastoraat als vorm van geestelijke verzorging in het moderne algemene ziekenhuis', in: *Praktische Theologie* 27 (2000) no 4, 365-374.

What do we understand spirituality and meaning to include?

As already mentioned in the introduction, this is a subject frequently far removed from the everyday problems that management in care institutions encounter. Budgets and their cuts, waiting and entrance times, the quality of medical care, negotiations with insurance companies, problems concerning research and teaching, personnel shortages, as well as many more issues demanding attention every day. The concepts of spirituality and meaning are moreover often so defined that managers can do little with them in practice.

Waaijman uses the concept 'divine-human transformation'; the 'divine-human' event of relationship considered from the angle of transformation.[4] Driebergen merely says that there should be attention to meaning and/or religion.[5] Van Leeuwen speaks of an integrating energy that is consciously or unconsciously present, causing mankind to experience meaning in his existence and be able to give meaning to it.[6] This integrating energy expresses itself in a personal way in the relationship with itself, others and possibly a higher being/God. Jochemsen *et al.* speak of spirituality in the functional sense, by which they mean: a manner of existence of all people and not only of people who subscribe to a certain religion.[7] They apply the following definition here: 'Spirituality is the ideological and religious functioning of mankind, to which the questions on the giving and experiencing of meaning also belong'.

As a point of departure for vision and policy we have chosen the following definition of spirituality: 'Both the patient and assistor in their relationship/interaction in health care are together guided by the giving of meaning, transcendence and/or religion as a fact of experience'.[8] The use of the term 'assistor' avoids making any statement on whether the professional medical and/or nursing assistor is intended or whether this involves a separate spiritual carer. We will return to this later.

Man is a spiritual being, able to give form and content to his or her life in a personal way. This is a fact that should be taken into consideration, in the

---

4 K. Waaijman, *Spirituality: Forms, foundations, methods*, Leuven 2002.

5 R. Driebergen, *Aandacht voor zingeving en/of religie: Verpleegkundige zorg op het gebied van spiritualiteit*, Groningen 2001.

6 R.R. van Leeuwen, *Zorg voor spiritualiteit, een verpleegkundig aandachtsgebied*, Maastricht 1997.

7 H. Jochemsen, M. Klaasse-Carpentier, B. Cusveller & A. van de Scheur, *Levensvragen in de stervensfase: Kwaliteit van spirituele zorg in de terminale palliatieve zorg vanuit patiëntenpersepctief*, Ede 2002, 12.

8 See also L.J. Tiesinga, J. Bouwer, H. Jochemsen, H. Blommestijn, K. Waaijman & D. Post, 'Spiritualiteit, (on)gezondheid en zorg: Een aanwezige en onderzoekbare relatie?', in: *Tijdschrift Sociale Geneeskunde* 80 (2002) no 8, 535-538.

provision of care too. Denial of this by some neither adds nor subtracts anything to this.

You may also choose another approach, as we find in Scheurich.[9] Spirituality belongs to religion, but it is so different to contemporary medical science that you have to keep these affairs separated from one another. The doctor should not deny spirituality, but keep himself at a distance, for he is not trained to deal with spiritual or religious questions. You cannot ask that of him/her either. It is true that spirituality and religion were close to each other in the past. In some non-western cultures this is still the case, but not in our Western culture. Moreover, this demands a kind of universally distributed belief from the population and this is no longer the case for us either. We agree on norms and values, OK, but prefer to keep our hands off other matters. The bio-psychosocial model in health care cannot serve as an excuse for the endless interference of health care in patients' personal life.[10] I feel this approach is incorrect, but it is attractive to management. I will return to this later.

Care for holistic care?

It is generally assumed that care stemming from a holistic vision of humanity will be the best care. This presumes that the somatic, spiritual, psychological and social dimension gets an equal degree of attention in the provision of care.[11] That the sum of co-operation between a somatologist, a spiritologist, a psychologist and a sociologist still does not deliver holistic care is, however, forgotten.

We see here the same misunderstanding that occurs in the so-called human modality therapy, the ill person is divided up into pieces, stomach, intestine, gallbladder, brains, etc. The sick part is treated; all the parts are reassembled and we have the whole person back, only now healed. It is a matter of integrating the different dimensions, which is more than co-operation. Moreover, it is a question hitherto unanswered whether *one* person should attend to all the dimensions or whether this ought to be four separate specialists.

Tiesinga et al. postulate that paying attention to meaning and/or religion not only contributes to the quality of care and the quality of life of the care seeker, but also to the quality of life of the caregiver.[12] It should be noted that not much

---

9 N. Scheurich, 'Reconsidering Spirituality and Medicine', in: *Academic Medicine* 78 (2003) no 4, 356-360.

10 Ibidem.

11 Tiesinga et al., 'Spiritualiteit, (on)gezondheid en zorg'.

12 Ibidem.

research has yet been done into the above mentioned proposition or hypothesis and that the evidence is therefore a little sparse. Everyone assumes that this is so, which is not the same as empirical proof.

Is the result better when treating a patient with an acute gallbladder inflammation if, in addition to a good surgeon, there is also someone attending to spirituality and meaning? Does a good surgeon suffice or should the surgeon do both? Opinions are divided on the question whether this and similar problems are even amenable to scientific study.

Yet it is important that more research, qualitative and if possible quantitative too, be done into this and comparable questions. If spiritual care-workers for example increasingly desire to position themselves as the professional colleagues of doctors, nurses and paramedics in care institutes, then one may also expect from them the same effort to underpin the correctness of their working methods with research.

Care perception of the institution

When the institution has formulated a perception of care, this should be carried out in practice by all of the institution's employees. How can management proceed in implementing this?

1. The perception of care can bear a prescriptive character. The management instructs employees to act explicitly according to this perception in their daily work. One does come across this in institutions tied to the church or having a strongly religious identity. Spiritual care-workers in such an institution are generally also members of the same religious domination to which the care institution is affiliated.
2. The perception may also be in the nature of guidelines. The perception is formulated in more general terms. The management leaves implementation of the perception to its employees. There is room for professional interpretation of the perception in practice, yet within a given framework. This is the preference of management of general institutions who do not want to advertise themselves as specifically committed ideologically (not especially as Roman Catholic, Dutch Reformed, Humanist, etc.).
3. For employees naturally have their own motivation for working in care too, and their own opinions about what is to be understood by good care. There is also room in the provision of care for individual interpretation of what motivates an employee in his or her life. Personal professional responsibility within a framework indicated by the management.

4. The perception of care can also be descriptive in nature. This contains a much greater freedom and even informality. The institution attempts to be as neutral as possible and desires to give its employees every opportunity of providing the care expressing their beliefs about what good care is. Regulations, universally accepted, statutory or laid down by the inspectorate, should be met. But above all, they should not be too specific.

In discussing these possibilities, a firm preference emerged for the second model. Both the responsibility of the institution as well as that of the individual professional practitioner would find its best expression in this model. The care seeker also gains the greatest freedom to ask for what he or she thinks is necessary in the area of religion and spirituality. 'Demand driving' is thus also possible on the patient's part.

Policy regarding assistors and assistance

Management may therefore instruct assistors to pay explicit attention to questions of spirituality and meaning making in an active, proffering sense. More passive and expectant action is also possible, and that far more attention might be implicitly given to questions of spirituality and meaning making.

Management may be of the opinion that providing integral care is a task for each individual assistor. Separate persons for specific spiritual care are then not necessary. Each carer pays attention to all aspects of care and the needs that she or he encounters in the caring and treating of patients. People should not only be educated in the technical aspects of assistance but also in giving attention to questions of spirituality and meaning.

In my view this option is as attractive as it is illusionary in our time. Each caregiver, with a few exceptions, has entered the profession intending to help people and not exclusively to treat intestinal cancer. We increasingly discover that we have to choose between aspects of total care. For providing integral care where there is attention to all that is necessary is quite impossible, simply due to lack of time. It seems to me to be an illusion to try to recreate this. Developments in medicine in the medical-technical sense are proceeding too quickly. Each individual assistor can try as much as possible to put this ideal into practice, but we cannot go much further and it is questionable whether this will yield very much.

Am I too sombre? I wish I were. The question arises regarding assistance as to how many 'preferences' management should offer. 'Something for everybody', so including ministers, Roman Catholic priests, Humanist counsellors, imams, pandits, winti and bono men, etc? A clergyman from every culture? Or should we keep to the denominations prevalent in our Western culture and try to have the others 'on call' (for example more than a hundred nationalities live in the Bijlmer in Amsterdam South-East, the AMC's catchment area)?

Should these spiritual carers be employed by the care institution or should there be institutes to train these people and then 'hire' them out to care institutions (so-called outsourcing)?

The spiritual carer may derive a certain authority from being connected to the institution: there is more continuity in care, the assistors know each other better and can also tailor the care better. Otherwise it would be a separate profession coming from outside and having little in common with the rest of the care provided. It also remains to be seen whether the patient is always going to feel like talking about spirituality and meaning on the appointed morning or afternoon. Management, however, has to realise that a team of spiritual care within the institution costs a lot of money and that budgets are increasingly under pressure. Diverse disciplines in health care have different ideas on the phenomenon of 'outsourcing' or employing spiritual carers.

A subsequent question concerns which patients are entitled to this assistance. The Quality Act has the 24-hour criterion. The number of spiritual carers is of such a nature that it is not possible to help every patient. How do we choose?

According to the above criterion, only the patients admitted to hospital for longer than 24 hours – clinical admissions and short stay patients – have a right to spiritual care. No spiritual care would therefore have to be offered for outpatient treatment, frequent outpatient care (being on chemotherapy drips for cancer for example), so-called 'peri-clinical' (day case) patients and patients already discharged, in transmural care for example.

In research into the need for spiritual care in periclinical patients it was apparent that this is clearly present. This concerns patients who although discharged from the clinic, must return for treatment to the hospital or outpatients so frequently that neither are they actually at home.[13]

It is difficult to quantify the need for care for these and other patients and it is still largely unrecognised. A chilly criterion of 24 hours does not seem adequate here. Research should begin into the care needs of the different patient categories we distinguish in modern medicine. Jochemsen et al made a start at this for palliative care.[14]

---

[13] De Vries & Van Gilst, *Kort dag.*

[14] Jochemsen et al., *Levensvragen in de stervensfase.*

The conclusion here was also that much is unknown and that there is much that is unquestionably accepted for which proof is lacking. Here too there is need of far more research.

In relation to the brief admittance times of the present day, management must answer the question on which priority should be given to the different types of care. Does care that is strictly medical always have priority in the scant time available? What balance in the provision of care should we attempt to find? Nowadays, there is not more time for all the things we might like. Is this good for the patient? Put up with it, get better soon, and just catch up with spiritual care at home later? An attractive option for tight budgets. But is this what we have chosen in these modern times or do we want to made a case for other, more balanced care which will then cost a little more?

These are all legitimate questions that naturally cannot be answered simply. Hopefully, the need for research will be increasingly understood, so that more data will become available and we can make more responsible choices.

A last but not unimportant question is: who is going to pay for all of this. Will the government do this? After all, it stated the requirement in the Quality Act. Will the health insurers do this, for example through the D (diagnosis) B (*behandeling*/ treatment) C (combination) system that is to be implemented?[15] Is it already included in hospital budgets as everyone, excepting of course the care institutions, would like to think? Is this the responsibility of organisations outside the institution: do they have to raise funds for spiritual care, for example via third party funding? Is it perhaps the responsibility of the collective churches in the catchment area for care institutions, as was the case for many years and still is in some parts of the country?

The importance of solving this problem is only intensified in the present climate of obligatory cut-backs and progressively tighter budgets for increasingly expensive care.

Developments in modern care institutions make holistic care ever more difficult

Finally we would like to pay attention to a number of developments in modern care institutions which make the giving of holistic care, if we should choose it, increasingly difficult. A number of these developments have already been considered above. We would like to briefly discuss a few things systematically. A

[15] DBC is the Dutch term for DRG (Diagnostic Related Groups).

few features of modern care institutions that might at the same time be termed developments are: (1) increasing influence of technology; (2) increase in scale; (3) pursuit of efficiency; (4) reduction of nursing time; (5) outpatient development; (6) transmuralisation (optimum co-ordination of intramural and extramural care); (7) increasing influence of legislation; (8) multi-culturalisation.

Increasing influence of technology

In recent decades, the emphasis in medicine has increasingly come to lie on technology. This has been fed by the explosive development of technical possibilities. Illnesses that not so long ago led to almost certain death can now be treated effectively – many forms of malign neoplasms (cancer), but also heart disease and infections for example. Focus and more emphasis on technology means less time for care. The word 'care institution' for a hospital has been replaced by 'treatment centre', which also reflects the character of the modern hospital better.

This trend to technology is also demonstrated in developments in the professions of specialists and nurses. There is specialisation and even super-specialisation within these professions. The patient often has difficulty in identifying the doctor, because treatment has become far more a task for a whole team. A result of this is the disappearance of the person as a whole entity in medicine. The sick person gives way to his sick parts and is also treated as if he were them. We speak of the person in terms of characteristics and parts anatomised by science and treat these modalities. We forget that the whole person is sick and so the whole person ought to be treated.

Now we definitely do not wish to deny that medicine's technical and scientific developments have been a blessing, on the contrary. But finding the correct balance in care for the whole person remains a challenge. This requires courage and ingenuity from workers in care.

Increase in scale

Many hospitals and other care institutions have fused in recent years. This escalating trend to the large-scale is dictated by the continuously rising costs of care. A large hospital is supposed to be able to work more efficiently and economically than a small hospital can. Even the use of the, often very expensive, equipment for diagnostics and treatment may be optimised in this way. The following step is extension of their operating time in order to use the machines more efficiently, and the wish to concentrate complicated and expensive diagnostics and treatment in specific centres. The power of technical control carries with it the danger of subordinating the human being, by ignoring specific spiritual-human values and characteristics. Of course this does not have to happen, but in my opinion there is too little attention paid to the danger of this at present. If priorities are to be considered, then attention to spirituality and meaning are way down on the list, if we do not keep a look out.

Pursuit of efficiency

Hospitals have been on a budget since the beginning of the eighties. Every year they are granted a sum from which care must be provided. It is not possible to do everything that one would like from this amount. Choices have to be made. The choices we make are usually in the medical-technical area. Care in nursing and care homes and institutions for disability care have meagre profit from this. Luckily there is growing interest in this problem, although as yet the extra monies apportioned to this type of care are only a drop in the ocean, given the serious arrears it has fallen into in recent years.

What the choices made are based on is often not clear either. On occasion the impression is created that the technical, the spectacular, that which attracts the most attention or the matters that have been promoted the best by patient associations are the things which profit the most. Real care is therefore underplayed. People who 'only need care' are not often heard. Here too is the advantage of technical achievements at the cost of other care; here once more is the challenge of finding a balance.

Reduction of nursing time

Hospital care is expensive, we have already seen this. One day of admission in an academic hospital costs more than one day of total care in the most expensive hotel in the Netherlands. Let us not mention the cost of a day in Intensive Care. It is therefore logical that in the context of efficiency and practicality it is attempted to limit patients' admission to as short a time as possible. The danger of catching hospital infections is also far less. Necessary examination is done in the out patient department as far as possible and only the most needful done on the ward itself: the treatment is done as well and rapidly as possible and then home or on to another form of care. During admission as good care as possible, but the emphasis should be first of all on the medical-technical aspect.

It is increasingly difficult for spiritual carers to find a moment for quiet conversation amongst all the examinations and treatments. The need for this is great and can only increase, for very radical things happen to a person in the hospital, far more than in the past. People are asked to make radical decisions in this age of increased independence, voluntary or obligatory. Within a very short period of time.

Equally, family and friends often understand very little of this. Here again the search for a balance between speed and efficiency, and the care of the whole person.

Outpatient development

As an extension of the above it is also logical that treatments are sought whereby admission to hospital for several days is no longer necessary. This has led to the development of outpatient departments and outpatient treatment (and also short stay wards): admitted in the morning, operated on immediately and home again in the afternoon. Of course precautionary measures are taken beforehand and there are all sorts of safety mechanisms built in to prevent anything going wrong for the patients. Again, emphasis on medical technology here, and to a far lesser degree on care. Indeed, there is no time for that, or hardly any. Moreover it is undeniably better for the patient to spend as little time as possible in the hospital.

Yet sometimes the very radical consequences of comparatively minor operations technically, demand a lot of a person's resistance. Taking a lymph node biopsy, even in the abdomen, is not the most difficult of medical interventions and may easily be done in outpatients. Yet the difference between a positive and a negative result, in the case of a malign tumour of the oesophagus or of the liver for example, means the difference between the possibility of an operation and treatment, and having to prepare yourself for death, perhaps within a few months. Certainty is quickly obtained, but what this signifies to a patient cannot be comprehended by healthy people who have never had to experience it.

Transmuralisation

When staying in hospital is no longer necessary but going home is not yet possible, connecting care outside the hospital is then sought for the patient. This might often involve further treatment in a revalidation clinic or temporary admission to a care home; sometimes home care or a visit from the district nurse. Sometimes permanent admission to a nursing home is necessary. Every effort is made to ensure that the pathway the patient takes may run as smoothly as possible, from the first visit to the GP to the hopefully healthy homecoming. This demands a lot of regulation, foresight and consultation with agencies outside the hospital.

A lot of care is devoted to this during admission and sometimes even before it. This is a good development for patients. The earlier you are home again the better, and if hospital is no longer the place for you, you had better be somewhere else to get the care that you now need.

A lot happens to a patient traversing such a pathway; usually he has scarcely had the time to realise what is occurring. Occasionally you hear in outpatients that a patient has needed a long time to come to terms with everything that has happened to him. Is this bad? In the end I don't think so. Nevertheless we must realise that although what we do is technically and objectively the best for the patient, it may still lead to psychological problems. People should be prepared for this and should be able to get help afterwards in processing things. That often seems to be very difficult.

Increasing influence of legalisation

The doctor-patient relationship is an unequal one, per definition. The doctor has knowledge, the patient has not. The doctor has power, the patient has not. The doctor is healthy, the patient is ill. In recent years health legislation in particular has sought to create legal measures giving the patient more rights vis-à-vis the doctor in legislation and regulations. A number of Acts, such as the Medicine Treatment Contracts Act (WGBO). The Care Institutions (Quality) Act and the Professions in Individual Health Care Act (BIG) are the results of this. The original doctor-patient relationship, typically a contact relationship, has increasingly become a so-called contract relationship. I am firmly of the opinion that the distance legislation was intended to bridge, has in fact increased. It would seem that doctor and patient safeguard themselves against each other through all sorts of regulations about rights and duties. It would be incorrect to blame legislation. Laws are a result of opinions and ways of thinking in society that have already existed for a longer time.

Then was it so much better in the past? Of course not! But a relationship of trust, by its very nature one of ethics, can not be replaced by a legal one without penalty. If, in the increasing speed and use of technology in health care, the basis of trust that there ought to be between doctor and patient is replaced by a treatment contract that is legally cobbled together, then the patient will suffer from it. This has never been the intention. Naturally, confidence in the doctor is not automatic because he or she is wearing a white coat. The attitude, performance and dignity of the doctor must earn it.

We increasingly see health care institutions take out cover, insuring themselves against patient claims. Patients also make complaints and claims to an increasing degree, often aided by lawyers who have made this their profession.

Naturally things happen that are not good, and people who suffer damage must of course be compensated. There ought, however, to be a better way of arranging this than by creating two opposing bulwarks of doctors and patients.

Multi-culturisation

A growing number of patients in our Dutch hospitals is of non-Dutch origin. Illness and disability is experienced and expressed in a completely different way and in a completely different cultural context. Dutch doctors and nurses will not have encountered this during their training. This is an increasing problem chiefly in those parts of the Netherlands where many immigrants settle, Amsterdam-South East for example. There are new challenges for spiritual care here too. Should it attempt to become more acquainted with these cultures or is more effective to incorporate imams, pandits, winti healers and bono men? We have mentioned this dilemma in this contribution before.

Conclusion

In addition to the many good things that modern medicine and the modern hospital bring us and which we should be thankful for, there are also developments containing a potential danger. We should all be prepared for these. The increasing influence of technology and legislation can promote dehumanising.

Increasing efficiency and practicality may lead to us losing our view of the sick person as a whole person, as a unique creation of God. If more and more time is necessary for technological action during a briefer and briefer working week and length of admission, there will be less and less time for care for the patient. The mission to love thy neighbour cannot only be interpreted in a medical technical sense, however important that part is.

The spiritual carer can fulfil an important role with respect to this danger of alienation between patient and doctor, in my opinion. For the patient he is someone who is indeed connected to the hospital, which lends him a certain authority. On the other hand he does have sufficient distance from the business of medicine to be the ideal person, a listening ear, to discuss things with peacefully, to consult for advice.

Guided by empathy and sympathy, the spiritual carer shows what it means to truly be a fellow human being. The feeling of having to be autonomous and independent can be cast aside for a while, to the relief of the patient. Many other questions and needs may be discussed in conversation with the spiritual carer, a human being just like the patient himself. A person is often confronted with his finiteness in an abrupt and harrowing way; business that has been pushed aside, perhaps for years, can no longer be avoided.

Even the spiritual carer often has no answer for many questions, something he has in common with the doctor by the way. Yet this may be amply compensated for by trust, presence, and intimacy in conversation, or sometimes merely by listening. Outlined in this way, I can only see increasing importance given to spiritual care in hospitals, and attention to spirituality and meaning. Management of care institutions should be aware of this and act on it.

As an essential part of health care, spiritual care can be an important part of 'the healing arts'. We doctors are often afraid that offering help and advice to a patient confronted with difficult choices, will quickly be seen as unacceptable paternalism.

Thus we are in danger of substituting the late Professor Rümke's advice to attempt 'a maximum approach with maintaining distance' in patient care, with 'a maximum distance due to fear of approach'.[16] For the distance can be minimal when we are truly moved by the fate of a fellow human being, which is preeminently the point of view of the spiritual carer. We obtain real quality in authentic care in this way.

On the other hand, the spiritual carer should be aware that he works in a professional environment and that he himself wishes to be seen as a professional. In our day and age, this includes attempting to objectify one's personal field of work and its results as much as possible through research.

BIBLIOGRAPHY

Bakker, D.J., 'Het algemene ziekenhuis van onze tijd: Pastoraat als vorm van geestelijke verzorging in het moderne algemene ziekenhuis' (The general hospital of our time: Pastoral care as form of spiritual care in the modern general hospital), in: *Praktische Theologie* 27 (2000), 365-374.

Driebergen, R., *Aandacht voor zingeving en/of religie: Verpleegkundige zorg op het gebied van spiritualiteit* (Attention to meaning making and/or religion: Nursing care in the area of spirituality), Groningen: Rijksuniversiteit Groningen, 2001.

Jochemsen, H, M. Klaasse-Carpentier, B. Cusveller & A. van de Scheur, *Levensvragen in de stervensfase: Kwaliteit van spirituele zorg in de terminale palliatieve zorg vanuit patiëntenpersepctief* (Vital questions in the terminal phase: Quality of spiritual care in terminal palliative care from the perspective of patients), Ede: Prof. Dr. G.A. Lindeboom Instituut, 2002.

16 H.C. Rümke, personal statement in a discussion with the author of this chapter.

Leeuwen, R.R. van, *Zorg voor spiritualiteit: Een verpleegkundig aandachtsgebied* (Care for spirituality: An area of attention for nurses), Maastricht: University of Maastricht, 1997.

Scheurich, N., 'Reconsidering spirituality and medicine', in: *Academic Medicine* 78 (2003) no 4, 356-360.

Tiesinga, L.J., J. Bouwer, H. Jochemsen, H. Blommestijn, K. Waaijman & D. Post, 'Spiritualiteit, (on)gezondheid en zorg: Een aanwezige en onderzoekbare relatie?' (Spirituality, health and the lack of it, and care: A present, researchable relationship?), in: *Tijdschrift Sociale Geneeskunde* 80 (2002) no 8, 535-538.

Vries, J.E. de & M. van Gilst, *Kort dag: Rapportage van de peiling Poliklinische Geestelijke Verzorging in het AMC*, Amsterdam: Dienst Geestelijke Verzorging AMC, 2001.

Waaijman, K., *Spirituality: Forms, foundations, methods*, Leuven etc.: Peeters, 2002.

IMPLEMENTATION

L.J. Tiesinga

SPIRITUALITY OF THE PROFESSIONAL IN HEALTH CARE

Spirituality is not only *in the air*, it is also to be found on the shop floor of ordinary health care. Nurses, doctors, or spiritual care providers all know situations where spiritual functioning – which includes questions of experiencing and making meaning – plays a role in care. This is not only about medically far-reaching decisions concerning life and death. It is equally about respect, attention and behaviour towards the patient. Spirituality is not only in intervention but also in presence. What is spirituality in health care? Which factors explain possible discrepancies in the spirituality experienced between patient and professionals, and that experienced between professionals themselves? Which questions may a professional employ as a guideline for analysing his or her own spirituality? These are questions central to this contribution.

First of all, naming various developments in health care introduces the theme of *spirituality of the professional in health care*, along with a description of relevant concepts, such as spirituality, health and care. A number of factors possibly explaining discrepancies in the spirituality experienced between the patient and professionals, and between the professionals themselves, are then named. These factors are placed in the context of health care, described in cases and analysed. Finally, a questionnaire for spiritual self-analysis is supplied. The professional can investigate what inspires and motivates him or her in the light of these questions. The factors described that may cause discrepancies in the spirituality experienced between professionals (and between professionals and patients) may be detected in this self-analysis. It is then possible for the professional to work on these inhibiting factors in practising care for spirituality.

What is spirituality in health care

Spirituality in health care seems to be a new phenomenon, yet it is not. Already in the Middle Ages people found inspiration in caritas when establishing hospices, places of worship and hospitals, and in caring for the sick. This can be traced back to diverse passages and stories from the bible and other holy books.

The parable of *The Good Samaritan* (Lk 10: 25-37) is perhaps the best known of these.

Although spirituality in health care is not a new phenomenon, the innovation of the present day is that spirituality – albeit on a limited scale – is integrated into care models and practices.[1] Practical theology, spiritual care provision, medical and care science have obviously rediscovered each other in this subject and that is beneficial. The rise of the scientific discipline of spirituality emphasises the relevance of integration and the object of study.[2]

In contrast to recent decades, we see an increase in interest in questions concerning multi-religious and non-religious spirituality. It would seem that religious spirituality has partly given way to non-religious spirituality. The content of the concept has thus shifted. Until recently it was primarily interpreted by caritas – charity and good works – with mercy as its source and inspired by biblical stories and symbols. Yet at present it is quite as applicable to non-religious outlooks on human beings and care. Anthropologically, spirituality may be termed '*the ideological and religious function of man, to which questions of giving and experiencing meaning also belong*'.[3]

In agreement with Van der Arend and Gastmans it may be stated that unlike ethical questions, spiritual questions are not directly related to norms and values.[4] The question for meaning is often central – who is man and what relationships does he maintain with his environment, nature and the Divine? Spirituality is more fundamental than ethics, and is the foundation of the norms and values driving our actions.[5]

1 WHO (http://www.who.int): WHO definition of palliative care, 2002; C. Gastmans, B. Dierckx de Casterle, & P. Schotmans, 'Nursing considered as moral practice: A philosophical-ethical interpretation of nursing', in: *Kennedy Institute of Ethics Journal* 8 (1998), 43-69; B. Neuman, *The Neuman systems model*, Norwalk 1995; J. Watson, *Nursing: Human science and human care, a theory of nursing*, New York 1988; M.A. Newman, *Health as expanding consciousness*, New York 1994; R.R. Parse, 'The human becoming theory', in: idem, *Illuminations: The human becoming theory in practice and research*, New York 1995; L.J. Tiesinga, R. Driebergen, & D. Post, 'Spiritualiteit en verplegen: Een literatuurstudie naar de plaats van spiritualiteit binnen het verpleegkundig kennis- en beroepsdomein', in: *Verpleegkunde* 18 (2003) no 3, 159-168.

2 K. Waaijman, *Spirituality: Forms, foundation, methods*, Leuven 2002.

3 H. Jochemsen, M. Klaasse-Carpentier, B. Cusveller, A. van der Scheur, & J. Bouwer, *Levensvragen in de stervensfase: Kwaliteit van spirituele zorg in de terminale palliatieve zorg vanuit patiëntenpersepctief*, Ede 2002, 12.

4 A. van der Arend, & C. Gastmans, *Ethisch zorg verlenen: Handboek voor de verpleegkundige beroepen*, Baarn 2002.

5 Ibidem.

Spirituality is being human and health is a process of becoming human, borne by a harmonious relationship between man and his human situation.[6] Not his or her illness, but man as a feeling, thinking and desiring being is central to Care. This attention to man's total physical, mental and spiritual functioning confirms the need for holistic, and so too spiritual, care.

After the Second World War, Dutch health care was transformed from a segregated, identity linked care and care institutions, into a general and non-identity linked care and care institutions. The management, scale enlargement, structure and financing of health care contributed to this.

The profession of spiritual caregiver has gained a place in Dutch care due to an updated professional standard with professional code, a concept registration system, legislation, financial assessment and by becoming embedded in organisations.[7] Although the spiritual caregiver specialises in spiritual care, this aspect of care fits the professional profile of other care professionals, including nurses and care attendants. Spiritual care is therefore not only an object of study for spiritual caregivers, but also for other assistors such as doctors and nurses.

The ideological and religious functioning of care professionals – to which the questions of giving and experiencing of meaning belong – does fit within the reflective and societal orientated competencies of the care provider.[8] To an increasing degree, care institutions are forced to develop their own identity and care outlook and to express it within organisation culture. This is due to social developments such as individualising, professionalising and the growth of cultures within Dutch society (Jewish, Christian, Humanist, Islamic, Buddhist, Hindu) on the one hand, and on the other the multidisciplinary approach to care.[9] These developments contribute to this renewed interest in spirituality.

To a greater or lesser degree, assistors have taken over care as we all know it in the case of illness or handicap. Assistors live with care. The consciousness of

---

[6] Kuiper, J., *Mensopvatting en gezondheidszorg*, Assen, 1980.

[7] Bouwer, J., *Van de kaart naar het gebied: Het domein van de geestelijke zorgverlening* (Inaugural speech Theological University of Kampen, Netherlands, 2003).

[8] B.S. Cusveller, 'De betekenis van levensbeschouwing voor verpleegkundige zorgverlening', in: *Verpleegkunde* 13 (1998) no 3, 149-157; R.R. van Leeuwen, & B.S. Cusveller, *Verpleegkundig competentieprofiel: Zorg voor spiritualiteit*, Ede 2002.

[9] L.J. Tiesinga, & D. Post, 'Spiritualiteit, who cares?', in: *Verpleegkunde* 17 (2002) no 2, 109-112.

that dependence and the demonstration of respect for the vulnerable fellow human being are – in dialogue with the other person – central values and fit the call for a more wholistic approach to care. Care is a form of being engaged in our world and in that of our fellow human beings with an eye to maintaining this world as well as possible.[10] Tronto distinguishes different care dimensions and attitudes to care. People may have cares about something (involvement), take on care (responsibility), carry out care (competencies) and receive care (receptivity). These dimensions of care can be applied to the aspect of spirituality. In care we are concerned with vulnerable and dependent fellow human beings.

In addition, a change is taking place in the approach to the patient and volunteer aid.[11] Care is increasingly aimed at the demand and needs of the patient and his or her helper in the community. In demand driven care, those involved investigate the needs of the patient and helpers and whether the nature, content, size, form, place and manner of care provision is attuned to what the individual patient requests or requires.[12] A cultural swing from offer driven care to need and demand driven care makes demands on the attitudes and competencies of the assistor – also in the field of spirituality. A recent development in the Netherlands is the appearance of a nursing competence profile with respect to care for spirituality.[13] It describes six competencies (see table 1). This profile might equally serve as a point of departure for other professionals in health care, such as for example the physiotherapist, behavioural therapist, social worker, GP, nursing home doctor and specialist.

In my opinion there is still discussion possible on this provisionally exploratory list of competencies in order to come arrive at adequate co-ordination with other disciplines. Factors will then be investigated which possibly cause discrepancies in the spirituality experienced between professionals, and patient and professional.

---

10 J.C. Tronto, *Moral boundaries: A political argument for an ethic of care*, New York 1993.

11 RVZ (Council for Public Health and Care), *Professionals in de gezondheidszorg*, Zoetermeer 2000; STG, *Een verzorgde toekomst: Toekomstscenario's voor verpleging en verzorging*, Utrecht 1997.

12 Platform Managed care and disease management, 'Disease management nog niet voldoende op de mens gericht', in: *HMF: Tijdschrift voor toekomstverkenning, strategieontwikkeling en innovatie* (special issue April 2001), 20.

13 Van Leeuwen & Cusveller, *Verpleegkundig competentieprofiel*; Idem, 'Naar een verpleegkundig competentieprofiel voor zorg voor spiritualiteit: Een verkennende literatuurstudie', in: *Verpleegkunde* 18 (2003) no 2, 72-81.

TABLE 1 COMPETENCIES OF NURSES[14]

1.	*The nurse can maintain own personal values, convictions and feelings in the relationship with care seekers with different ideologies* • Show respect for the ideology of the care seeker: unprejudiced towards people, churches and schools of thought about life • Reflect on the exchange between personal spirituality (values and convictions) and the reactions that the care given or received arouse in her; for example feelings of powerlessness, sadness, fear of illness, suffering, death and the influence of personal experiences • Be open to other interpretations than her own, prevent the pathologising of spirituality, prevent the forcing of her own ideology on the care seeker • Recognise and acknowledge personal boundaries in dealing with the care seeker's spirituality and express this with respect to the care seeker and in the team • Refer to another caregiver adequately and in time (for example colleague or spiritual carer)
2.	*The nurse can communicate with care seekers from different cultures about their spirituality in a concerned way* • actively listen to aspects of the 'ordinary' spirituality of the care seeker and to spiritual aspects in relationship to his illness/handicap • accept the other, is involved, sympathetic, gives confidence, is empathetic, real, sensitive, sincere, selfless, close, touches, applies relevant conversation techniques (taking care of the care seeker's reaction to bad news and aspects of transcultural communication among other things)
3.	*The nurse can collect information about the care seeker's spirituality and determine care requirements in conversation with that care seeker* • Collect, order and clarify information on 'ordinary' spirituality: ideological background, religious biography, the life story, significance of mystical and religious experiences, use, rituals, symbols and traditions in daily life • Ask and/or observe what is the influence/significance of the care seeker's own spirituality on experiencing and coping with the illness/handicap and what influence/significance the illness/handicap has on that spirituality (among other things spotting non-verbal behaviour and symbol language) • Use of measuring instruments/questionnaires for a spiritual assessment • Can determine the spiritual care requirement of the care seeker and formulate it in writing
4.	*The nurse can in conversation with the care seeker and consultation with other disciplines co-ordinate care for the care seeker's spirituality and plan and record in writing his/her own part in the careé* • Report both verbally and in writing on the care seeker's spiritual functioning (care requirements, planning, realisation and evaluation) and be concerned about continuity in the care for spirituality

[14] Van Leeuwen & Cusveller, *Verpleegkundig competentieprofiel*; Idem, 'Naar een verpleegkundig competentieprofiel…'.

	• Report both verbally and in writing on the care seeker's spiritual functioning (care requirements, planning, realisation and evaluation) and be concerned about continuity in the care for spirituality • Estimate who can best give the necessary care for the care seeker's spirituality • If desired, transfer care for spirituality to a nurse with the same convictions as the care seeker • Refer the care seeker if desired to a spiritual carer (for questions on faith and/or about life, performing rituals) and see to it that the contact is made – if necessary consulting a spiritual carer on questions about the spiritual guidance of the carer
5.	*The nurse can carry out care for the spirituality of the care seeker and evaluate that care in conversation with the care seeker and in multi-disciplinary consultation* • Help the care seeker in continuing spiritual customs ('ordinary' spirituality) such as rituals, prayer, meditation, reading, music, or carry out these for the care seeker • Give information about facilities in the institution (spiritual care on offer, meditation centre, services among other things) • Attention to spirituality in providing basic care to the care seeker (among other things climate/atmosphere in ward, in physical care, daily rituals) • Pay attention in conversations with the care seeker to thoughts and/or feelings that bring to mind handicap, illness, suffering or death • Discuss questions on life and meaning with the care seeker against the background of his/her life story (among other things fear and insecurity, putting life into perspective, clarifying outlook on life, naming incongruities, supporting the process of assimilation, help in deciding, supporting self-acceptance, resilience, rounding off goal/balance in life, dealing with death wish/euthanasia request, stimulate to talk with others) • Offer hope and consolation (among other things questions as to future plans, helping setting goals, is realistic, encouraging pleasure in the everyday, using good moments) • Employing relaxation exercises and complementary interventions • If necessary, guidance of family/friends in the field of spirituality (among other things information on facilities in the institution, such as spiritual care on offer, guidance in communication with the care seeker, attention to their own feelings/thoughts) • In conversation with the care seeker check whether there has been sufficient attention to the care seeker's story in the provision of care, whether the request for spiritual care has been posed correctly and whether the care has been well adjusted to it
6.	*The nurse makes a contribution to the quality of care and advancement of expertise in the area of care for spirituality within the care institution* • Raises the issue of work problems in the area of care for spirituality to care seekers in supervision discussions and coaches other care providers in this area • Makes recommendations to management about care for spirituality • Carries out improvement projects in the area of care for spirituality

Which factors explain possible discrepancies in the spirituality experienced between professionals, and professionals and patients?

These factors will be described in the light of cases and analyses detecting possible discrepancies in the spirituality experienced between professionals and patients. The factors are sometimes difficult to separate but can be differentiated. The factors are reproduced in diagram form in table 2.

TABLE 2 FACTORS THAT MAY EXPLAIN DISCREPANCIES IN THE SPIRITUALITY EXPERIENCED BETWEEN PROFESSIONS, PROFESSIONALS AND PATIENTS

1.	Life orientation: difference in life orientation
2.	Time orientation: difference in experiencing time
3.	Place orientation: difference in experiencing place
4.	Person orientation: difference in experiencing person
5.	Treatment orientation: difference in orientation to treatment
6.	Quality of life: difference in experiencing quality of life
7.	Engagement: difference in involvement with each other in care
8.	Responsibility: difference in responsibility in care
9.	Competence: difference in competencies in care
10.	Receptivity: difference in 'being receptive' in care
11.	Research model: difference in theoretical frameworks
12.	Research method: difference in research methods
13.	Philosophy of science paradigms: difference in philosophy of science frameworks

1. Life orientation – case and analysis

Four cancer patients lie in a ward in a general hospital. Although therapeutic treatment has commenced, they all know that they are incurably ill. One patient is Muslim, another patient is Hindu and the other two patients are humanists. The background of one of the nurses that day is Christian, another is humanist. The specialist treating them is Jewish.

During the specialist and nurses' round, where the patients are discussed individually, a discussion occurs in the patients' room. The patients with a religious background find it very disagreeable that there is so little space and opportunity for silence and prayer. They would like to pray to God a lot, in order to assimilate their illness and situation and to be able to fully address what is to come. The other patients need conversation and a lot of people visiting them. This disturbs other people's rest. The patients with a humanist background do not understand what these religious patients mean by a Hereafter – for them after death things are finished and done with. Their needs are still primarily for conversations with family, friends and acquaintances. The nurses do not know what to do about this. The specialist is a religious person himself and understands the wish of the religious patients, but also understands that it cannot always be peaceful. The end of the story is that the religious patients desiring a lot of silence for prayer and meditation are put in a separate room, to their great satisfaction.

Analysis: A different outlook on life causes life and death to be viewed in a different way. That means that a difference in way of acting, experiencing and culture often occurs. It should be made explicitly clear in the provision of care that the philosophy of life of patient and professionals is an issue needing ongoing attention.

2. Time orientation – case and analysis

At the end of her day shift, a nurse drops in to see a patient on a ward of a general hospital. She would have liked to go on talking to the patient earlier in the day but nothing came of it because of pressure of work on the ward. The patient heard yesterday that no further medical treatment is possible for him and that he has a bad prognosis. The specialist has told him that he has a few more months to live. After the nurse has talked with the patient for half an hour, she lets him know that she has to round off the conversation. She has another appointment to play tennis with a friend. Just as she wishes to leave the sickroom, the specialist attending him appears. He wants to keep up to date with the situation. There is a multi-disciplinary consultation planned for tomorrow at which the patient will be discussed. After five minutes the specialist leaves too – he feels he can do no more for the patient, and time is money. The patient looks at his clock. Isn't time a strange concept, he thinks. Earthly life is limited by death. One person gets to be 88 and another 5. From the point of view of his faith in eternity, however, there is no longer a limit on time in his perception. This does make his earthly time – however brief – still important. He makes a decision to make the best of the time he has left.

Analysis: The nurse primarily experiences her time as being within the context of daytime duty. She is available for care in that period. Finiteness does not play a direct role for her. How different for the patient. He has been told he only has a few months to live. Time for him gains a completely different meaning – due to the limit that has been set to it. For the patient, finiteness and eternity play an important role in his care. The specialist is subject to strict planning, expressed in units of time. High density of information costs less time and so less money and increases the income.

3. Place orientation – case and analysis

The situation takes place in a pavilion for mentally handicapped people in the grounds of an institution. In the day time the residents work within a sheltered workshop. After the evening meal the residents are happy that they are allowed do their own thing. Three days ago a new supervisor started work. She is married and has three children. She lives in a detached house with a lot of room. Another supervisor lives by himself. Another one lives with a partner. Most of the residents like music very much – only not all of them like the same kind. The residents have been arguing for more self-sufficient spaces in the pavilion for some time, for example a separate bedroom for every resident. This has been without result up until now. The residents have to share the rooms. One resident loves gospel music, another heavy hard rock.

Analysis: During their work the group supervisors are in a place which is home to the residents. The supervisors come and go and can withdraw to their homes for peace. The residents already have to take the other residents far more into account – as well as visitors and suchlike. In spite of this they have no room for themselves.

4. Person orientation – case and analysis

The situation takes place in a rehabilitation centre. A CVA patient is admitted for lengthy rehabilitation. The rehabilitation doctor treats the patient and co-ordinates this with other professionals. The patient's family is closely involved with the treatment and there is contact with fellow sufferers. The professionals and the care seekers each have their own role and complement each other.

Analysis: Different people participate in the care process. Those giving and seeking care are central. Each caregiver ascribes a separate professional role to himself. The difference in roles lead to completely different ways of being occupied with care: care receiver, fellow-sufferer, volunteer carer, minister/priest, practitioner, therapist, supervisor, carer.

5. Treatment orientation – case and analysis

A patient is admitted to a general hospital for a liver transplant. This drastic operation has been discussed beforehand with the specialist attending him. The specialist, together with a nurse, briefly pops in to see the patient again the evening before the operation takes place. Once arrived in his room the patient expresses the wish that the spiritual carer say a prayer together with the medical team. The specialist does not think this belongs to his repertoire of treatments and takes no notice. The nurse proposes consulting the spiritual carer. On the same evening the spiritual carer says a prayer together with the patient – without the other professionals involved.

Analysis: The diverse professionals involved in caring all have their own vision of the treatment. The specialist does not feel called to participate in an activity of the pastor. In this case, the spiritual care provider takes no part in the multidisciplinary consultation, while this would be most desirable.

6. Quality of life – case and analysis

On an IC ward in a general hospital a terminal patient is given oxygen and is continuously checked with the aid of monitors. In view of the patient's terminal situation and the possibility of also being cared for at home with the aid of extramural care, the family requests that their mother's intramural medical treatment be ended. One of the family's arguments for taking their mother home is that in their opinion her quality of life will increase, however relative. This wish is finally granted. Once at home the patient dies three weeks later.

Analysis: The various parties – patient, volunteer carers and professionals – look at quality of life in different ways. For the doctor, the medical view point of worthwhile or not worthwhile medical treatment is paramount. Others would perhaps allow other arguments to count, such as rest, social and spiritual support from volunteer care.

7. Engagement – case and analysis

A nurse works on the children's ward of a hospital. When she walks into a child's room she comes across a mother of a child admitted with leukaemia praying on the ground. The woman is Moslem and was just then occupied in doing her morning prayers at sunrise. She tells the nurse how important the prayer is for her and that she firmly believes that it works. The nurse – herself a humanist – does not really understand what the woman means but respects her opinion. She becomes more involved with the woman's conduct because of her story. By chance the child's specialist drops by during the coffee break. He says a little nonchalantly that it mustn't get any crazier. Now the parents want to pray with their child in the room five times a day. We can't start that, you know. The nurse says that she has more understanding for this – and in the end succeeds in convincing the specialist that it is very important for the woman. The nurse feels very involved with the situation and gets to know the woman better and better. That the woman does her prayers in her child's room five times a day becomes more and more normal.

Analysis: Not everyone is equally involved with the patient and his or her family. For most of the time nurses are present in the ward during their work.

They often build up a relationship with the patient and the family. Because of this they generally have more eye for and attention to non-medical affairs than for example medical specialists or other professionals in care.

8. Responsibility – case and analysis

An 88 year old patient in bad physical condition and admitted to a somatic nursing home has let the team treating him know that he wants to go on a pilgrimage to Lourdes once more. A volunteer carer of the patient is prepared to go there with him. It is difficult for the multidisciplinary consultation to take a decision. The nursing home doctor considers it to be medically irresponsible that he should go. Given his physical condition – serious degree of chronic heart failure and regular physical symptoms such as dizziness and very high blood pressure – the desired undertaking might have fatal consequences. The nurses on the other hand say this desire might be important for the patient, particularly at this time.

Analysis: In this case it is difficult to come to a decision. Medical responsibility lies with the doctor. Treatment as a whole is a responsibility of the team. The patient and volunteer care have their own responsibilities here.

9. Competencies – case and analysis

The family of a Catholic patient in the ward of a general hospital let a nurse know that their mother has indicated that she wishes to receive extreme unction. The nurse answers that she will consult the spiritual care provider. The specialist in attendance is consulted as well. The medical specialist says that this activity is outside his competence and passes on the question to the spiritual care provider. The spiritual care provider who visits the patient lets him know that he shall consult a Catholic colleague about administering extreme unction. As a non-Catholic spiritual care provider she is in fact not judged competent to administer extreme unction.

Analysis: Extreme unction may only be performed by a competent Catholic care provider. Other professions are not competent to be allowed to carry out this procedure.

10. Receptivity – case and analysis

A patient is admitted to a psychiatric institution. During the case history it becomes clear that the patient has many depressive symptoms stemming from guilt feelings. The patient seeks the cause in his perception of religion. According to the patient he has committed a sin that cannot be forgiven. In his view he is condemned to hell. He feels very downcast because of this. The psychiatrist, who is also religious himself, takes these feelings into account and involves them in treatment. The patient is happy about this because this means a lot to him. The nurses on the ward also observe symptoms that could have something to do with the religious life of the patient. The nurses take this aspect of the patient seriously and report their observations and findings in the patient dossier.

Analysis: Both the psychiatrist and the nursing personnel show respect for the religious life of the patient. They are receptive to information the patient supplies in this area and the patient himself is also receptive to care in this area.

11. Research model – case and analysis

A cardiology patient is discussed during a multidisciplinary consultation in a revalidation centre. The cardiologist in attendance is chairman of the team. On the basis of research and observation it has been determined that the patient suffers from chronic heart failure and that heart rehabilitation is desirable. The case is mainly discussed from the standpoint of the medical model. Medical parameters are extensively argued. Psycho-social aspects of the illness are merely mentioned at best. The spiritual caregiver who does not take the sickness but the sick person as point of departure, gains no entry into the medical debate. Little is done about proposed activities in the spiritual sphere.

Analysis: Spiritual care providers do not think in medical jargon and yet other disciplines again have their own concepts and models. Art and skill will be needed to design a model whereby the sick person in addition to medical diagnosis and treatment will be discussed in an interdisciplinary, integrated way from the perspective of patients.

12. Research method – case and analysis

During a congress on 'soul, illness and care' two research assistants presented their doctoral degree research. One tries to interpret the bible text of the Good Samaritan with the aid of the structure analytic method. A feature of this approach is that the researcher assumes the autonomy of the text. The other PhD student has developed a theory of 'involved care' with the aid of the *grounded theory*-method. After the discussion, the researchers begin conversing with each other. This turns out to be unfruitful as the conversations run aground because neither understands the other one's applied method.

Analysis The PhD students assume different methods of research. This often makes scientific debate between the disciplines more difficult on the meta-level. Disciplines often know far too little of the methods of the diverse schools and traditions to be able to carry out a good debate on them.

13. Philosophy of science – case and analysis

During a symposium, two professors enter into conversation with each other about their view of sickness and health. One professor of spirituality attempts to give insight into what it means to be confronted with AIDS at a young age. The images he uses are powerful and fit within the language field of the humanities. The other professor of social medicine backs up his arguments using completely different language. His arguments are tangibly and empirically established. He makes use of statistics and experimental research.

Analysis: There are various approaches to reality in scholarship. A lot of linguistic and hermeneutic research occurs in the humanities. Much attention goes to understanding and getting the feeling of things. In contrast, the social and medical sciences serve a more empirical approach. It is aimed at gaining knowledge based on observation and experiment. Both academic approaches utilise another language field. The art is to understand both, and not to make one superior to the other.

In summary, a number of factors are described which may illucidate the discrepancies in the spirituality experienced among and between professionals and patient. Empirical research will have to demonstrate whether in addition to the factors mentioned there are still other factors influencing the spiritual dysfunction of and the relationship among and between professionals and patient. The following paragraph will specifically explore the spiritual functioning of the professional.

In what way can a professional investigate what inspires and hinders him or her?

Work in care. It would seem to be self evident – yet it is not. The fact of the matter is that working as a professional in care demands inspiration and passion. Passion, in order to guide and care for individuals, pairs and families in case of illness, suffering, infirmity, and death. This goes further than a formal work relationship and touches people personally.

In addition, it is presumed that attention to spirituality makes a contribution to the quality of care. The quality of care improves if assistors have space in their work for their own spirituality.[15]

---

[15] L.J. Tiesinga, J. Bouwer, H. Jochemsen, H. Blommestijn, K. Waaijman, & D. Post, 'Spiritualiteit, (on)gezondheid en zorg: Een aanwezige en onderzoekbare relatie?', in: *Tijdschrift voor Gezondheidswetenschappen* 80 (2002) no 8, 535-538; L.J. Tiesinga, & D. Post, 'Het spiritueel functioneren van zorgvragers en zorgverleners in de gezondheidszorg: Een synthese', in: *Verpleegkunde* 18 (2003) no 4, 272-278.

On the basis of personal values and motivations or possibly for other reasons – whether conscious or not – professionals choose to work in the care sector. They confront themselves in that care. Whether a professional works as a nurse, carer, nursing home doctor, GP, medical specialist or spiritual carer, the questions of meaning and inspiration keep on bobbing up and demanding that they be deeply considered. This can be pleasurable but frustrating in equal measure. For example reflection on work may cast light on the fact that a discrepancy exists between desirability and reality. It is important that professionals are then conscious of this and can possibly work on improvements. Attention to spirituality is important where the quality of care is concerned, whether professionals have just started work or whether they are even very advanced in the work process.

This spiritual self-analysis gives a professional the opportunity to investigate what gets him or her moving, how he or she gets moving, how he or she stays moving (at work), and where work can still be done. The analysis is aimed at the person participating actively and contributing examples, trying to be conscious of the place and position that he or she occupies in spiritual care. This spiritual self-analysis is reproduced as a diagram in table 3.

TABLE 3 SPIRITUAL SELF-ANALYSIS

What sets me in motion?

- What are my sources of inspiration?
- Am I inspired by certain persons, near by or far away, from the past or in the present?
- Am I inspired by nature?
- Am I inspired by certain animals or things?
- Am I inspired by certain writings?
- Am I inspired by meditation or prayer?
- Am I inspired by certain works of art?
- Am I inspired by certain values?
- Are there any other sources that inspire me?

What gets me moving?

- Which way leads me to get moving?
- Do I get moving because of rational analysis and considerations?
- Do I get moving because of social-emotional experiences?
- Do I get moving because of acting upon things?
- Do I get moving because of spiritual experiences?
- Are there any other ways leading me into movement?
- How do these aspects influence each other?

How do I stay moving?
- What keeps me moving?
- How do I maintain my spirituality?
- In what way do I stay in contact with my sources of inspiration?
- How can I make a place for them there?
- How can I take time for them there?
- How can I give that shape?
- What do I have to do or not do?

How do I stay moving at my work?
- What is the link between my own spirituality and the work that I do?
- What motivates me to work in health care?
- What way leads me to do my work in health care?
- How do I maintain my spirituality in relationship to my work in health care?

What do I still have to work on?
- What stimulates or inhibits me from harmonising my work with my own spirituality?
- Why do these factors stimulate or inhibit me?
- Is there anything to be done?
- Can I do anything?
- How can I do anything about it?
- How can I learn to deal with it better?

To summarise: it may be stated that, through self-analysis, the professional can investigate whether, in what way and to what degree spirituality plays a role in his or her life and work. This self-analysis can contribute to consciousness of sources of inspiration and the experiencing of spirituality. The experiencing of spirituality in meeting the vulnerable sick person is not seldom a motivation to work, and remain working, in care. To prevent burn out and demotivation is therefore extremely important that professionals continue to pay attention to their spiritual functioning. Optimum spiritual functioning of professionals will contribute to the quality of care.

Summary

Questions about the spirituality of the professional in health care are best answered from the point of view of a practical situation, because of conceptual diversity. The functional and practice-directed description of spirituality given by Jochemsen *et al.*[16] – where man as an anthropological being is central – can serve for this: *man's ideological and religious functioning, to which questions of giving and experiencing meaning also belong.* Man's ideological and religious functioning differentiates itself from somatic, psychological and social functioning,

[16] Jochemsen et al., *Levensvragen in de stervensfase*, 12.

but is not separate from it. Indeed, man's spiritual functioning is directly connected to somatic, psychological and social functioning. Someone may directly foster his or her spirituality in prayer, meditation or dance for example by assuming a specific physical attitude, by encouraging a psychological state, or by placing himself in a certain social context. On the other hand, man's spiritual functioning equally influences his or her somatic, psychic and social functioning. Man's spiritual functioning has thus a reciprocal and direct relationship with man's somatic, psychological and social functioning.

The importance of the professional's spiritual functioning is still insufficiently recognised in health care. Although there are initiatives demonstrating that spiritual care in health care and research into this phenomenon is increasingly important. Examples of this are the design of a competence profile for nurses,[17] the compilation of a list of nursing interventions in the realm of spiritual care[18] and the founding of RESPIRE (*Working Group of Research in the field of Spirituality-Health-Care*). In the light of spiritual self-analysis, the professional would be able to investigate what gets him or her moving, how he or she gets moving, how he or she remains moving (at work), and what he or she can still do to improve – possibly under the supervision of a specialist in the field of spiritual functioning in care. A spiritual self-analysis is supplied in this article, which professionals in care might use for themselves.

Diverse factors may play a role in the creation of discrepancies in the spirituality experienced among professionals, and between them and their patients in health care. The question is rather what factors these are, and in what way and direction and to what degree do they have influence. A number of factors imagined to be relevant are described in this article, illustrated by cases. Although a series of factors are introduced, the question as to whether all relevant factors have been detected has not yet been answered. Exploratory and empirical research into the spiritual functioning of professionals in health care will have to throw light on this.

A word of gratitude

My thanks go to Annemarie Tiesinga-van der Lijn for her comments on the first version of this manuscript.

---

[17] Van Leeuwen & Cusveller, 'Naar een verpleegkundig competentieprofiel…'.

[18] R. Driebergen, L.J. Tiesinga, & J. Bouwer, *Aandacht voor zingeving en/of religie: Verpleegkundige zorg op het gebied van spiritualiteit. Delphi-onderzoek naar een verpleegkundige interventie* (Presentation at the Flemish-Dutch scientific congress: 'Evidence based practiced: the present state of affairs', Antwerpen, 14 December 2001), Abstract.

BIBLIOGRAPHY

Arend, A. van der & C. Gastmans, *Ethisch zorg verlenen: Handboek voor de verpleegkundige beroepen* (Giving ethical care: Manual for the nursing professions), Baarn: HB, 2002.

Bouwer, J., *Van de kaart naar het gebied: Het domein van de geestelijke zorgverlening* (From the map to the district; the domain of spirital care provision), Inaugural speech Theological University of Kampen, Netherlands, 2003 (Kamper Oraties no.24).

Cusveller, B.S., 'De betekenis van levensbeschouwing voor verpleegkundige zorgverlening' (The significance of philosophy of life for nursing care provision), in: *Verpleegkunde* 13 (1998) no.3, 149-157.

Driebergen, R., L.J. Tiesinga & J. Bouwer, *Aandacht voor zingeving en/of religie: Verpleegkundige zorg op het gebied van spiritualiteit. Delphi-onderzoek naar een verpleegkundige interventie* (Attention to meaning and/or religion: Nursing care in the area of spirituality. Delphi research into a nursing intervention), Presentation at the Flemish-Dutch scientific congress: 'Evidence based practiced: the present state of affairs', Antwerpen, 14 December 2001. Abstract.

Gastmans, C., B. Dierckx de Casterle & P. Schotmans, 'Nursing considered as moral practice: A philosophical-ethical interpretation of nursing', in: *Kennedy Institute of Ethics Journal* 8 (1998), 43-69.

Jochemsen, H, M. Klaasse-Carpentier, B. Cusveller, A. van der Scheur & J. Bouwer, *Levensvragen in de stervensfase: Kwaliteit van spirituele zorg in de terminale palliatieve zorg vanuit patiëntenpersepctief* (Vital questions in the terminal phase: Quality of spiritual care in terminal palliative care from the perspective of patients), Ede: Prof. Dr. G.A. Lindeboom Instituut, 2002 (report no.16).

Kuiper, J.P., *Mensopvatting en gezondheidszorg* (Human outlook and health care), Assen: Van Gorcum, 1980.

Leeuwen, R.R. van & B.S. Cusveller, *Verpleegkundig competentieprofiel: Zorg voor spiritualiteit* (Nursing competence profile: Care for spirituality), Ede: Prof.dr.G.A. Lindeboom Instituut, 2002 (report n. 17).

Leeuwen, R.R. van & B.S. Cusveller, 'Naar een verpleegkundig competentieprofiel voor zorg voor spiritualiteit: Een verkennende literatuurstudie' (Towards a nursing competence profile for care for spirituality: An exploratory literature study), in: *Verpleegkunde* 18 (2003) no.2, 72-81.

Neuman, B., *The Neuman systems model*, Norwalk: Appleton and Lange, 1995.

Newman, M.A., *Health as expanding consciousness*, New York: National League for Nursing Press, 1994.

Parse, R.R., 'The human becoming theory', in: idem, *Illuminations: The human becoming theory in practice and research*, New York: National League for Nursing Press, 1995.

Platform Managed Care and Disease Management, 'Disease management nog niet voldoende op de mens gericht' (Disease management not yet sufficiently focussed on the human being), in: *HMF: Tijdschrift voor toekomstverkenning, strategieontwikkeling en innovatie* (Magazine for futurology, strategy development and innovation), special issue April 2001, 20-22.

RVZ (Council for Public Health and Care), *Professionals in de gezondheidszorg* (Professionals in health care), Zoetermeer 2000.

STG (Council for Future Explorations in Health Care), *Een verzorgde toekomst: Toekomstscenario's voor verpleging en verzorging* (A cared for future: Future scenarios for nurses and care), Utrecht: Tijdstroom, 1997.

Tiesinga, L.J. & D. Post, 'Spiritualiteit, who cares?', in: *Verpleegkunde* 17 (2002) no 2, 109-112.

Tiesinga, L.J. & D. Post, 'Het spiritueel functioneren van zorgvragers en zorgverleners in de gezondheidszorg: Een synthese' (The spiritual functioning of care seekers and caregivers in health care: a synthesis), in: *Verpleegkunde* 18 (2003) no 4, 272-278.

Tiesinga, L.J., J. Bouwer, H. Jochemsen, H. Blommestijn, K. Waaijman & D. Post, 'Spiritualiteit, (on)gezondheid en zorg: Een aanwezige en onderzoekbare relatie?' (Spirituality, health and the lack of it, and care: A present, researchable relationship?), in: *Tijdschrift voor Gezondheidswetenschappen* 80 (2002) no 8, 535-538.

Tiesinga, L.J., R. Driebergen & D. Post, 'Spiritualiteit en verplegen: Een literatuurstudie naar de plaats van spiritualiteit binnen het verpleegkundig kennis- en beroepsdomein' (Spirituality and nursing: A literature study into the place of spirituality within the field of nursing knowledge and profession), in: *Verpleegkunde* (Nursing) 18 (2003) no 3, 159-168.

Tronto, J.C., *Moral boundaries: A political argument for an ethic of care*, New York: Routledge, 1993.

Waaijman, K., *Spirituality: Forms, foundation, methods*, Leuven: Peeters, 2002.

Watson, J., *Nursing: Human science and human care, a theory of nursing*, New York: National League for Nursing, 1988.

WHO (http://www.who.int): WHO definition of palliative care.

F.W.J. GRIBNAU & M.A.M. PIJNENBURG

SPIRITUALITY AND MEANING IN CARE
AGENDA POINTS FOR CARE INSTITUTIONS' QUALITY POLICY

Tradition, belle lettres and the visual arts all tell a tale: that the place of care, in the literal sense of location, is a very special one. A legacy has accumulated here, the most essential in human existence is present, in its experience and deeds, in the environment and actions of human communities, in the lives of individuals asking for and providing care. For example, a legacy may be discovered in Jorwerd, the presence of one who is a non-Absentee. One of the authors (FG) struck up a conversation with an inhabitant of Friesland while taking a holiday snapshot of the place-name sign for Jorwerd. He intended it to serve as a bookmark for the book 'How God disappeared from Jorwerd' by the Dutch author Geert Mak.[1] In that conversation, during which much was said, he was allowed to note down the man's words: 'I have to get this off my chest. Of course God is not gone from Jorwerd. There are a couple of reasons why. In the first place God has not left Jorwerd, because God never leaves anywhere. We Dutch people might think that, or an important writer might think it, but God just doesn't ever leave somewhere. Moreover, if He ever felt inclined for a moment to leave, then my wife, our two sons and I would definitely call him back every day, because we happen to pray daily before our main meal. That is the second reason. And thirdly – and now I'm thinking of the Christian loving God who encourages we human beings to be the Good Samaritan – just look at that farm there. A woman has been lying there sick for years. If you could see how she's cared for! God is not gone from Jorwerd'. The inhabitant involved, needless to say, thought the title of this book about the soullessness of the little place appropriate, but *also* had to tell about the above.

[1] Jorwerd has set many people thinking. The dean of the Nijmegen faculty of Theology at that time made a theme of the subject during an international anniversary symposium. Gerard Rooijakkers also treated *How God Disappeared*, as the case may be, from Jorwerd in: J. Bluyssen & G. Rooijakkers, *God verborgen en nabij: Religie als heilig spel* (God hidden and nearby: Religion as holy game), Amsterdam: Anthos, 2002, 159-165.

Introduction

In recent decades, spirituality and meaning have been treated stepmotherly in care institutions. For a long time questions concerning meaning, inspiration, soulfulness and cohesion were regarded as primarily personal matters, shared with friends or trusted conversation partners, if desired. It was policy in care institutions to organisationally 'regulate' attention to this type of question into a separate service of spiritual care, or pastoral service. There are great questions of direction that are of importance in care institutions – strategies for the future, medical planning, conditions of employment, demand driven care etc. Yet for these questions spirituality and meaning remained marginal areas, not really relevant to what was going on.

Since the beginning of the nineties it has been felt increasingly clearly within the Radboud University Nijmegen Medical Center (UMC St Radboud) that such questions concerned are that vital that they ought to be part of quality policy. In this contribution we will briefly investigate some background circumstances of this choice and the way in which the choice is worked out, using a familiar quality cycle: plan, do, check and act.

A few background circumstances

For many a healthy citizen, disease or threatened health are considered questions that well-equipped instances tackle, curb, preferably solve. Where it serves a purpose they even go along with the maxim 'you ask – we do'. Good equipment includes guaranteed, up-to-date professional and organisational quality, borne by an attitude of service and compassion. In the year 2003, guarantees are required to combat possible fragmentation in the realisation of such quality, due to the use of part-timers who are very differentiated in function. Moreover the actual interaction between those seeking and those offering care is burdened by a rather unsettled conceptual framework: Notions such as: 'market conformity' or 'free choice', for example, turn out to be hollow phrases where vital questions are concerned. In less threatening situations, they are opportunities or reasons for lapsing into inessentials. But to all appearances the average Dutchman has every reason to feel positive: we live in a prosperous country, if you like, a prosperous and safe province of Europe. The efforts of many dedicated and resourceful, capable forces will enable much good and increasingly better care to be given to an increasing number of people in need of care, and there is no reason to assume that this will change drastically.

Yet, there are also signs of disturbance and unease. Patients and healthy people show concern about possible mistakes and failures. Doctors are becoming sombre: for many, their dream of the medical profession has turned into a nightmare, due to pressure of the work among other things. Those in training suffer from stress.[2] Costs are mounting, or rather, resources increasingly and very obviously turn out to be finite; we seem to be on the verge of a divide. Complementary medicine is flourishing disproportionately. Use of anti-depressants is growing substantially. There are major concerns about the syndrome of dementia. Catch-up measures are necessary to counteract the erosions of previous policy. Budgeting, for example, has been exchanged for the market mechanism of supply and demand and its accompanying jargon: consumer and suppliers, competition and rivalry, care as a product of cost effectiveness and calculated quality. At the same time, there is trepidation that this sort of trendy language, however needful in itself, is at odds with care.

But there more is involved: the finiteness of human life and even its cessation arouse great ethical and spiritual questions. It is discomforting to observe in our Western culture a public image of man where, on the one hand, the autonomous individual is central, and rightly so. While on the other hand, essential dimensions of human existence – the physical, psychosocial and meaning giving or spiritual being – no longer have, or no longer seem to have, any connection with each other. The question as to 'living meaningfully' often seems to be asked in the life of an individual when he is in sight of his approaching end. This happens possibly even more frequently nowadays. There is talk of a general loss of memory and meaning in Western society and individuals. It has grown and it is still growing, so that knowledge of one's own moral sources has run dry and an existential peril and fear of meaninglessness is left.[3]

Against this fear of meaninglessness, enough public spirit exists that dares to speak of both a shared image of man and of togetherness. This public spirit exists among those working in the caring profession, among those who train for it and among countless volunteer carers. Growing globalisation likewise rectifies the one-sidedness of this Western public image of man. Happily, globalization does not only work to lower barriers with respect to anti-terrorism measures, but also offers every opportunity of contact with the countless inhabitants of the Earth for whom social existence (as a healthy or sick person) and religious life are not essentially different quantities. For these people only know one life, the human in all its aspects.

This summary sketch should suffice to make the following proposition defensible. That at this juncture, the policy agenda of institutions, umbrella

---

[2] D. Pendleton & J. King, 'Values and leadership', in: *British Medical Journal* 325 (2002), 1352-1355.

[3] Ch. Taylor, *De malaise van de moderniteit* (The malaise of modernity), Kampen: Kok Agora/Kapellen: Pelckmans, 2000 (11th ed.; orig. publ. 1991).

organisations, and society may, and indeed must, concern itself with the soul of persons, businesses and institutes as a duty, as a right, even as a privilege or priority if you like. Care Institutions should pay attention to the aspects of care and the maintenance of the soul on their policy agendas. They should be part of policy and plainly mentioned by name. This should not look like a lurch to the right or to past centuries in a secularised world that is evidently no longer understood.

The soul, point of departure for quality policy

The preceding description might be also valid as a report of a 1992-1993 exploration conducted within the Radboud University Nijmegen Medical Center.[4] for the purposes of a chapter on 'Identity and Ethics'. This was for a strategic policy plan to be formulated for 1995-2000. All departments in our house were consulted under a central direction. The word 'privilege' was also mentioned at this time, for care institutions may be compared with roundabouts or traffic art installations on the life paths of those seeking and providing care. Many a time the real questions about routes through life operate here – whether we want them to or not. The following minutes were taken at a work conference 'AZN and Medical Ethics':

> The AZN wishes to express 'in clear language' the 'great values' in a well-considered and balanced way where important matters, such as life and death, are concerned.

It was considered a logical necessity to first explore the dimension of ethics – the good self, the good life and good acting – and its limits. In addition, feelings of alienation in dealing with the question involving the meaning of human life were expressed. It was also noted:

> In the world of care, the human mind, body [such coordinate severance is in itself an intolerable dichotomy] *and* the soul are never really lost to each other, at most losing sight of each other on occasion.

A number of things resulted in a special area of attention for policy and organisation: spirituality and meaning. This was further elaborated below, in the auto-evaluating and reporting manner customary for a quality inspection. Our report consists of four parts, corresponding to the terms of a frequently utilised blueprint for quality assurance: 'plan, do, check, act', or rather the so-called 'PDCA cycle'. This PDCA blueprint partly does justice to personal experience, but is at the same time intended to take some distance to it, in order to avoid the appearance of well-

---

[4] Before the fusion of the Faculty of Medicine and the Academic Hospital in 2000 its name was AZN: Academisch Ziekenhuis Nijmegen St Radboud.

meaning ego-tripping. We intend to work on thinking about, even preparing, a policy translatable into steps according to everyone's state, scale and situation.

Briefly specified the PDAC cycle runs as follows:

1. Thought, PLAN – before
2. tackle – DO, in action
3. then occasionally scratch one's head – CHECK, revision,
4. and afterwards proceed refreshed – ACT, on course?!

The management of an institution may thus operate without being pedantic or manipulative, although a suspicion or danger of this may lurk in those areas. For those involved, a votum of assurance is fitting for this approach. We quote from John's letters 3:18 and 24: 'My little children, let us not love in word, neither in tongue; but in deed and truth. And he that keepeth his commandments dwelleth in him, and he in him. And hereby we know that he abideth in us, by the Spirit which he hath given us'.[5]

1. PLAN, after hearing, briefing

The following quote is from our institution's strategic plan for 1995-2000 mentioned above, which is published and distributed under the title *Academic Profile Creation*

> Regarding moral questions, the AZN first of all realises that it functions in a pluriform, multi-cultural and multi-racial society within which many philosophies of life and religions are present.
> AZN chooses a position from the point of view of its own responsibility. It allows itself be guided by evangelical insights and norms, and their interpretation by the Church authorities and by the Catholic community in the Netherlands, as well as by opinions and beliefs current in Dutch society as a whole.
> The AZN deploys essential points of departure such as care and carefulness in the approach to patients. It realises that compared to other hospitals it is not exceptional in this.

The Hospital policy plan is founded on a clearly formulated identity:

> The AZN has its roots in the Catholic population. From the position of a Catholic academic hospital in a pluriform society, the AZN chooses for clear involvement of Catholicism in its vision and standpoint with respect for and in dialogue with other beliefs.[6]

---

5 Willibrord Translation, 's Hertogenbosch: Catholic Bible Foundation, 1995.

6 AZN St Radboud, *Academisch profileren: Strategisch beleidsplan van het Academisch Ziekenhuis Nijmegen St Radboud 1995-2000* (An academic profile: Strategic policy plan of the Academic Hospital Ziekenhuis), Nijmegen: St Radboud, 1995, citations on p. 17.

All this was not intended to be a mission statement in the sense of a fashionable 'must', it was definitely intended to be written down and implemented in deeds. Our PLAN encompassed good, generally comprehensible and widespread expressions of principles, prior to and underlying a number of well-chosen actions.

We expressly did not select a plan to broadly research the place and significance of religion in the institution, although it is quite conceivable that we might have done so. T. Schepens collected facts of this order in 1983-1984 among institutions that were members of the Christian Association of Care Institutions (CVZ); this formed the basis of its later Tilburg dissertation.[7] We chose – here responding to demand – the development of education for our own employees, touching on questions of meaning per department. It was a form of 'supportive contemplation' concerning the soul of their lives and professions, dwelling on what they experienced as part of their being, relating the self to the most important of all or possibly The Most Important. In Christian terminology this may be termed as the relationship between creation and Creator, between God and his child.

The KVZ[8] of the time assumed the role of setting up schooling, and taking care of associated reporting, also in the sense of offering other institutions what we had learned from experience. The commission was defined as a project, with a broader formulated project target:

> To help develop the leading role of the AZN St Radboud with respect to promoting and giving tangible content to ethical contemplation and policy within Catholic institutions. The AZN St Radboud considers that it has a special responsibility in this area, given its position as the only Catholic academic hospital in the country.

The project got the name 'agency', due to its representative task of propagating, and where necessary giving account for the visions and positions of the AZN St Radboud concerning ethical and identity related questions.

---

7 Th. Schepens, *Plaats en betekenis van de godsdienst in Christelijke ziekenhuizen: Een sociologisch onderzoek bij ziekenhuisorganisaties en bij het verplegend en verzorgend personeel* (Place and significance of religion in Christian hospitals: A sociological research into hospital organisatons and into nursing and caring staff), Tilburg: Tilburg University Press, 1997.

8 KVZ: Catholic Association of Care Institutions, founded in 1976. Hospitals, nursing homes, institutions for mentally handicapped, care homes and institutions for mental healthcare are among the roughtly 120 institutional members. Against the background of its Catholic identity the KVZ furnished contributions to social debate on the policy and course of care and about ethical themes.In addition, it provided education in the field of ethics, philosophy of life, identity and meaning making. In 2003, the KVZ fused with the Christian Association of Care Institutions (CVZ). This association has similar aims and activities and operated against the background of a Protestant identity. The new association founded in 2003 still bears the name 'CVZKVZ'.

The feasibility of the above mentioned training on questions of meaning was researched as a pilot in a few wards – neurosurgery, plastic surgery and geriatrics. The training was comprised of three evenings in co-operation with teachers from the Spiritual and Pastoral Care Service, the Titus Brandsma Institute in Nijmegen and professional peer supervisors. The results of these pilots were positive: the training appeared workable and was welcomed as good and valuable. The fact that this training was offered by the management of the institution in the first instance and subsequently also encouraged, belonged to the PLAN phase.

When opportunities arose where the central requirement was to act well ethically, the training directed itself to practical and methodical instruction and preparation in case directed moral deliberations in clinical wards. Here, the so-called 'Nijmegen Method for Moral Deliberation' was introduced and deployed as a blueprint for thought and reasoning.[9]

In 1997, a steering and adjoining support committee was started for the more detailed planning and guidance of the project. It included persons with a medical, nursing, pastoral and management background, under the chairmanship of a member of the Board of Directors. The Secretary was Mr M. Pijnenburg, general secretary of the KVZ and co-ordinator of the agency project. After a while the group gave itself a name relating to its programme: Adviescommissie Levensbeschouwing en Ethics op de Agenda – ALEA (Advice Commission Ethics and Philosophy of Life on the Agenda). This name indicated that the ALEA did not want to linger in profound considerations about identity, but wished, given the Catholic identity of the hospital, to address itself to the question of which tangible efforts and activities this should and could lead to. It did and does, however, see itself as a supportive think tank for research into Catholic or Christian identity. This is viewed thematically as one of the identities forming modern pluralistic culture, and also as one of the sources of meaning in modern culture (with reference to the Canadian philosopher Charles Taylor.[10] In 2004-2005 there will be more detailed publication on this research by the Department of Ethics, Philosophy and History of Medicine from the Radboud University Nijmegen Medical Center to be abbreviated as Department EFG.

---

9 See for a description: N. Steinkamp & I. Uerz, 'De Nijmeegse methode voor moreel beraad op de werkvloer' (The Nijmegen method for moral advice on the shop floor), in: M. Pijnenburg & M. Nuy (Eds.), *Abstineren: Morele overwegingen bij het staken van levensverlengend medisch handelen* (Abstaining: Moral deliberations on ceasing life extending medical treatment), Budel: Damon, 2002, 17-23.

10 Among other things: *Sources of the self: The making of modern identity*, Cambridge: Cambridge University Press, 1989. A clear introduction of Taylor's view is presented in: I. Breuer, *Taylor: Kopstukken filosofie* (Top people in philosophy), Rotterdam: Lemniscaat, 2002.

2. DO: in action, turn the intended into deeds

Under the supervision and management of the ALEA, the points of departure and work appointments named and written down in the first part were subsequently realised. In the course of 2002, an internal report was published on the activities performed.[11] Some facts and points of evaluation from it follow.

- After the pilots mentioned above, the training on offer was named 'Meaning and Care'. It was utilised by a range of categorical, multi-professional teams (clinics for mouth/jaw surgery and ear, nose and throat; cardiology; the coronary care unit; both our day case and health care centre medical oncology teams). Participants received a certificate of participation. They indicated that they had experienced the short course, followed by several peer supervisions as inspiring, exceptional, enlightening, and also too short. Doctors were under-represented among the participants. One keyword from the evaluation made, appeared to have noteworthy value as a word: mercy. This word often came across as loaded, sometimes dangerous, also sometimes dangerously old-fashioned. Students, teachers and supervisor recommended that this and other communication regarding questions of meaning, care and professionalism should be made more widely available.
- Training and follow-up training also took place in the region. There, four institutions had decided on more intensive collaboration a number of years ago. They called themselves by the abbreviation CARS, referring to the former names of Canisius-Wilhelmina Hospital, Academic Hospital Nijmegen, Rijnstate Hospital and St Maartens Clinic. CARS has a commission for projected training courses, among other things. This commission arranges a course in ethics for assistant physicians in training, provided by the EFG department.
- The ALEA was one of the initiators of the so-called Prudentia project. This consists of an annual congress concerning an actual question of ethics in hospital practice, partly illustrated from the Catholic perspective, and as a result of which a publication is issued. This project was initially realised along with Flemish speaking Belgian partners, and after that with a group of six Dutch hospitals. The themes were: 'Value judgements and conflicts of conscience in health care'; 'To treat and not te treat in medicine';[12]

[11] M. Pijnenburg, *Eindverslag Agency-project UMC St Radboud-Katholieke Vereniging van Zorginstellingen (KVZ) 1997-2001* (Final report Agency project Radboud University Nijmegen Medical Center – Catholic Association of Care Institutions), Nijmegen-Den Bosch, 2002.

[12] Publications of the same name, under editorship of M.Pijnenburg, published privately, resp. 1999 and 2000.

'Abstaining';[13] 'The hospital as moral community';[14] 'Aggression in the hospital'[15] and 'Dying from multicultural perspective in the hosptial'.[16] The conferences attracted an average participation of around 90 persons, coming from hospitals over the whole country and from various disciplines.

- Moral case deliberations in the ward gained a regular place in a number of clinical departments. This deliberation is a systematic and methodic interdisciplinary discussion of morally problematic case histories. It began in the mid-eighties as hospital-wide evening meetings entitled 'Ethics on the shop floor'. In the nineties, it developed towards case deliberations in wards, partly as a component of the PLAN phase mentioned above. Latterly, the EFG department has also given courses on moral deliberation, outside the Radboud University Nijmegen Medical Center in care institutions in the Netherlands and Germany. The KVZ was also active in this area.
- Compared to other universities, the EFG department makes a substantial contribution to the education of doctors in the field of ethics and, partly because of its position within a Catholic Radboud University Nijmegen Medical Center, selects its main points of research from the fields of palliative care and genetics.
- The Radboud University Nijmegen Medical Center has gone public on two other, important occasions. First of all, at the centenary of the Geneeskundige Vereniging ter Bevordering van het Ziekenhuiswezen (Medical Association for Promotion of the Hospital System). This was founded by physician directors, who put medicine first before directorship. Deliberations concerning material and existential finiteness were made in an article and during a symposium.[17] Moreover on the occasion of the millennium, the Catholic and Christian Association for Care Institutions and the Raboud University Nijmegen Medical Center organised the congress 'Chosen for care: a challenging legacy'. This congress attracted a great deal of attention and is remembered by many as a joyful and worth-

---

13 Pijnenburg & Nuy, *Abstineren*, 17-23.

14 M. Pijnenburg & M. Nuy (Eds), *Het ziekenhuis als morele gemeenschap* (The hospital as a moral community), Budel: Damon, 2003.

15 M. Pijnenburg & M. Nuy (Eds), *Agressie in het ziekenhuis* (Aggression in the hospital), Budel: Damon, 2005.

16 M. Pijnenburg & C. Leget (Eds), *Multicultureel sterven in het ziekenhuis* (Dying from multicultural perspective in the hospital), Budel: Damon, 2006.

17 F.W.J. Gribnau & M.A.M. Pijnenburg (2000), 'Eindigheid als perspectief, eens in de eeuw of...' (Finiteness as perspective, once in the century or...), in: *ZM-magazine* 16 (2000) no 12, 3-7.

while occasion. Hundreds of religious sisters, brothers and deaconesses were guests of honour. The congress was a expression of gratitude to them, for their works of foundation and expansion relating to present Dutch healthcare and geriatric care. This gratitude took the form of treating the question of how their legacy could be fruitful both for today and tomorrow. The diagnosis was that questions of meaning and spirituality are often no longer structurally anchored in current care, but nonetheless inevitably present themselves over and over again. It is characteristic of our culture, however, that such questions are often marginalised and are primarily viewed as individual matters. The congress and the subsequent report book[18] published helped care institutions present their own positions in a distinctive way. In this, they offered room for existing or redefined identity, for the relationship between meaning and care, between inspiration and professionalism as the heart of the quality of care.

- Two important pieces of the care institution's standard equipment for both its primary task and for the reflection which remains necessary, is of course the Pastoral Service and the Ethics Commitee. They must be actually visible and not just speak or be spoken of in the organisation chart and the annual report. To do this, they deserve to gain the means and not just be facilities for particular occasions. They should not be at the bottom of the list. They should therefore be equipped for their task, *and* held responsible for it. Then their policy proposals do form important advice. Management should test whether their preliminary advice fits into the organisation, and afterwards make its decision.
- At more special moments, we must give attention to what we should just summarise as 'transcendence': in New Year Speeches, in addresses on the occasion of departure or anniversaries. An appropriate special moment for illustrating this transcendence is always the introduction day for new employees. In a welcome word from the Board of Directors, the question 'Why are we here? Why do we do...?' is posed in order to greet the newcomers in a committed, professional way. The commitment expected of them in turn is seen as fruitful inspiration. Our most recent logo is the dove, referring to the Holy Ghost from the logo of the Radboud University Nijmegen, with the seven gifts of the Spirit radiating from its wings like beams. Since its introduction, these seven rays have been mentioned here: wisdom, insight, counsel, strength, knowledge, piety, and awe of

[18] M.A.M. Pijnenburg & P. van Mansum (Eds.), *Voor zorg gekozen: Een uitdagende erfenis. Bundel naar aanleiding van gelijknamig congres, 30 maart 2000* (Chosen for care: A challenging legacy. Collection from congress of same name), s.l.: CVZKVZ-UMC St Radboud Nijmegen (privately published).

God. In the discussions after such a word of welcome, a first move not infrequently leads to follow-up conversation, quite often in the hospital corridor or bike shed afterwards.

It should be clear that which is outlined above is not mentioned because of its robustness, but because of its possible exemplary benefit. Each institution can – and perhaps must – translate questions of meaning and spirituality into deeds, with an explicit approach and availing itself of opportunity. An example of such an occasion, utilised by the management, was the attempt to fuse Centrum De Poort and the Vondelstede care home in Amsterdam without 'losing your face'. As PLAN-DO phase of quality assurance regarding the 'Face', member of the board H. Kuiphof described guarantees for preventing identity problems with fusions.[19]

3. CHECK: review, on course?

The third term from the language of quality assurance is 'check': the test of what has been done up until the date set and at the same time the prelude to continuation, adjustment or fundamental review. The initial balance drawn up of what has been accomplished renders the following picture:

- As already described, training is available in the field of questions of meaning, initially offered in a highly top-down manner, with the assumption that there is need for this. The range on offer and the content of the training is directly linked to the practice of executing one's professional duties. The training is noted as important by the Board of Directors, so should be followed in the employer's time, and reinforced by a certificate of participation. After a few years experience and on the basis of evaluations, it has turned out that not only is such a course 'acceptable', but also desirable, fully-booked: it is thought a 'must'. At the moment, even departments are indicating that they would like to follow this course.
- There is a great deal of activity in the area of ethical reflection and questions. There are moral deliberations in the clinic, Prudentia, the integrated place of ethics in education and research, activities in collaboration with and on behalf of other institutions. This activity does not work out in rapid, sweeping changes, but rather in 'mustard seed strength'.
- Contributions to a centennial party or millennium event hit the mark. They remain in many people's memory for a long time and put time-honoured questions onto the agenda again: about the place and significance

[19] H. Kuiphof, 'Hoe bewaren wij ons gezicht: Waarborging voorkomt identiteitsproblemen bij fusies' (How do we keep our face: Guaranteeing prevents identity problems on fusion), in: *ZorgVisie* (Views on Care) 26 (1996) no 12, 20-24.

of human finiteness within a medicine that increasingly promises to prolong the length of our life. Or about the hunger for a contemporary, not fashionable, but authentic spirituality of care.

The check likewise serves as an upbeat for how we should proceed. We have already said it, on mustard seed power: a sense of reality is suitable, rapid and flashy successes are not guaranteed, failures are also possible. Reality forces a few sober conclusions:

- The attempt at multi-disciplinarity in schooling, for example demands targeted recruitment among the medical staff inviting them to participate, or offering another form of involvement.
- The workload, unmistakably increasing, prompts many a roster planner to be reserved about all kinds of matters that are immediately necessary; attention to spirituality and meaning can then rapidly turn into a minor consideration.
- Insofar that the legacy of Christianity obtains specific attention, there should be ellucidation – the involvement of the Radboud University Nijmegen Medical Center in this determines the way it carries out its task.[20]
- Continuity for the annual open event with a theme is a substantial task, as is carrying out policy concerning philosophy of life and identity.
- Not every year is a centennial, let alone a millennium. New reasons must be sought.

Care institutions are secular institutions, or already were, or have become so. On this point there is no difference between care institutions with a confessed, formulated religious identity, Catholic for example, and institutions that do not interpret their identity in this manner. The secular character of care institutions likewise offers them room to call themselves Catholic at the institutional level, and at the same time give employees and patients the freedom to choose their own source of life. Within the actual pluralism of philosophy of life movements, a shared, and for a care institution vital, pattern of values is very possible indeed. But religion and meaning also arise within pluralistic environments. They are not phenomena that merely occur in so called 'identity based institutes' but belong to the reality of the human experience itself. As a comparison, when we replace 'Union' with 'care institution' in one sentence of the concept of the European Constitution, you may read:

---

[20] See Strategisch Beleidsplan (Strategic Policy plan) UMC St Radboud, *Koers op kennis – kennis op koers* (Course in knowledge – Knowledge on course), Nijmegen 2002, 8.

> The values of the care institution, our care institution, contain both the value of those who believe in God as the source of truth, justice, goodness and beauty, and of those who do not share this belief but respect these universal values as deriving from another source.

This is not new, even for believers, for the Gospel did and does not claim exclusive rights – thank goodness. An even more important indicator for the place of philosophy of life and meaning than a debate about whether to name Christianity in the Constitution of Europe, is a statement from the World Health Organisation WHO. This was made in the Christmas number of the *British Medical Journal*.[21]

> The World Health Organisation reports: Until recently the health professions have largely followed a medical model, which seeks to treat patients by focusing on medicines and surgery, and gives less importance to beliefs and to faith – in healing, in the physician and in the doctor-patient relationship. This reductionist or mechanistic view of patients is no longer satisfactory. Patients and physicians have begun to realise the value of elements such as faith, hope and compassion in the healing process.

The columnist of the British Medical Journal editorial concerned noted the following under the subtitle 'Spiritual values and skills are increasingly recognised as necessary aspects of clinical care':

> Many see religion and medicine as peripheral to each other, yet spirituality and clinical care belong together.

It should be obvious: demand for spirituality arises from the sickbed and from the experiences in and around the sickbed.

The score to date reproduced here in a few lines justifies continuation of the course of the policy. The word 'course' is used here deliberately because the Radboud University Nijmegen Medical Center chose the title 'Course on Knowledge – Knowledge on Course' for its new strategic policy plan, dated February 2002. It describes the three core tasks of our university medical centre: transfer of knowledge, knowledge development and knowledge application. This new policy plan, including the sections concerning mission, identity, questions of meaning and culture, arose from intensive institution-wide consultation within the organisation.

One finding of the members of the NIAZ[22] team who thoroughly inspected our institution for accreditation, was observed absence of connections between a trio of commissions in our house: the Ethics Committee, the Committee on

---

21 L. Culliford, 'Spirituality and clinical care', in: *British Medical Journal* 325 (2002), 1434-1435; also to be seen in relationship to: P. Kohnen (Ed.), *Euthanasia and human dignity: A collection of contributions by the Dutch Catholic bishops*, Leuven: Peeters, 2002.

22 NIAZ = Nederlands Instituut voor Accreditatie van Ziekenhuizen (Dutch Institute for Accreditation of Hospitals).

Research involving Human Subjects and the Guidance Commission Prenatal Diagnostics and Therapy. Furthermore, they concluded that the strategic choice of moral deliberation in the department was not anchored at cluster level, the level of our divisions. These findings of sharp-eyed, well-prepared outsiders summon us to learn and act upon them. In other words, the accreditation process furnished at least one policy advice worthy of consideration: 'Allow yourself to be inspected'.

PLAN, DO and CHECK contributed to the following identity paragraph in the new strategic policy plan:

> The UMC Radboud has its origins in the Catholic community of faith and wishes to carry out the tasks it stands for with commitment and specific attention to its spiritual legacy. The UMC Radboud realises that it functions within a pluriform, multicultural society. Based on this understanding, the UMC expressly takes responsibility for itself, and has respect for and is in dialogue with other beliefs.
> The Christian humanitarian tradition within the UMC St Radboud is translated in various ways. Tender thoughtfulness is a guiding notion in patient care, which may be particularly found in special attention to pain control, palliative care and chronic illnesses. The idea of solidarity is reflected in the historically close contacts with various Third World countries. This leads to intensive education exchange, whereby Nijmegen students of Medicine do internships as medical students in the Tropics, and Third World doctors follow courses of education in the UMC. Scientific research into tropical disease has also had a long tradition within the UMC.
> Its ideological roots ensure that the UMC pays a lot of attention to medical ethics. Ethical standpoints, prepared by the Ethics Committee, are published both in the scientific and general media.
> The 'moral deliberation in the ward offers individual employees a platform where questions of meaning and moral questions come up for consideration. Prepared by the 'Adviescommissie Levensbeschouwing en Ethiek op de Agenda' (Advice commission Ethics and Philosophy of life on the Agenda), this deliberation has already rendered much good experience in a few wards. The intention is to obtain wider acceptance for this initiative. The activities outlined, allied to the identity of the UMC, are witness to the fact that the UMC does not only shape its function as a top knowledge centre through knowledge, transference and the application of advanced medical knowledge. The understanding is present that when eye to eye with human needs balancing on the border between life and death, medical technology knows its limitations and knows that top care may also signify abstaining from further medical intervention.[23]

[23] See Strategisch Beleidsplan UMC St Radboud, *Koers op kennis – kennis op koers*, 8-9.

4. ACT, on course...?!

Then the last of the four quality terms: ACT, proceed refreshed, on course?! After a quality inspection and an awarded accreditation, an action plan should be clear and brief, with reference to the accredited positions. It is therefore logical to briefly introduce the obvious next steps, which are commissions. The ALEA fulfils a driving, stimulating role for many of the actions mentioned below.

- First of all, the changeover from top-down to bottom-up. An empirical research was started in 2003 into the informal identity, as a basis for outlook development on giving shape to the formal identity, institutionally anchored. A questionnaire was developed through interviews and theory, constituting an instrument for quantitative research among roughly a thousand participants. Research results are expected in the course of 2006.
- Keep using events to set and to maintain questions of spirituality and meaning on the agenda. One of the events utilised involved the farewell symposium for our former dean, Prof. Vooijs, under the title: 'Good Work, contribute to discussion on quality in healthcare'. The introductory remarks to this symposium approached quality from the dimensions of philosophical ethics (Prof. Dr. P. van Tongeren), spirituality (Prof. Dr. C. Waaijman) and medical experience (Prof. Dr. C. Moolenaar).
- Increasing participation and involvement of physicians, in consultation with the clinical staff convention. This is particularly requested for an exceptional area of work that is developing, that of palliative care.
- Management makes itself responsible for doing its utmost not to give low priority to what has now been put on the agenda with respect to spirituality and meaning. Naturally one must not go so far as to be unreasonable and unfair: one must make the most of finite human power and means.
- In consultation with the institution inspectorate, raise the matter of some formation expansion on behalf of the recognised 'big job', even in times of scarcity.
- Increase of familiarity, knowledge and skill in areas such as the formation of conscience,[24] professional ethics[25] and the doctrine of virtues.[26]
- Active interpretation of the membership of the Reliëf.

---

[24] *Katechismus van de Katholieke Kerk* (Catechism of the Catholic Church), Brussels: Licap, 2005, f.i. p. 390, §1778: 'Het geweten is de eerste van alle plaatsbekleders van Christus'. (Conscience is first of all the Vicars of Christ).

[25] J. Dupont & C. Hermans, *De beroepsethiek van fysiotherapeuten en HBO-verpleegkundigen* (The professional ethics of physiotherapists and academic nurses), Budel: Damon, 2001.

[26] P. van Tongeren, *Deugdelijk leven: Een inleiding in de deugdethiek* (Virtuous living: An introduction to the ethics of virtue), Amsterdam: SUN, 2003.

- Active participation in the challenging, enriching forums which religious contacts offer nationally and internationally.[27]

Incomplete – Safely on the way

In the above, spirituality and meaning were approached as questions of policy and organisation. To this end we have utilised a handle from the social sector of quality control. A characteristic of quality assurance, however, is that this is never allowed to boast of completion. The characteristic of never being finished belongs to the essential core of quality, thus one continually asks anew: what is quality here and now? Quality is entrusted to us, forming and reforming it is a constant commission.

Identity does not allow itself to be regulated in essence but develops in relationship between individual people. Christian identity as commission is a 'verb': it encourages continual effort to connect inspiration with the way in which core tasks are performed. This connects to the quality policy of an institution.

The inspiration for the UMC St Radboud flows from a source of faith, which recognises as criterion the dignity of each person as one of God's creations. It puts emphasis on a brotherly and sisterly community of people, and trusts in a meaningful reality (although not always experienced as such). This reality is the motivation for seeking meaning and relationship in human experiences and undertakings.[28]

---

[27] M. Pijnenburg, 'Identiteit steeds belangrijker in katholieke gezondheidszorg: Vat (congres Pauselijke Raad voor het pastoraat in de gezondheidszorg en AISAC, Rome, November 2002)' (Identity is increasingly important in Catholic health care: Congress Papal Council for pastoral care in healthcare and AISAC), in: *Een-twee-een* 30 (2002) no 19, 667-678.

[28] Many activities are also undertaken by others in the area of seeking meaning and connection. A few examples:
KVWZ, *Vormingsgids identiteit en levensbeschouwing* (Guide to forming Identity and philosophy of life) Loose leaf overview of courses and supervision, collected by the then association together with PVO, 1995; M. Steemers-Van Winkoop, *Geloven in zorg: Omgaan met geloof, levensbeschouwing, spiritualiteit in de gezondheidszorg* (Belief in care: Coping with faith, philosophy of life, spirituality in healthcare), Baarn 2001; G. Danneels, *Is een oude honger terug? Schoonheid als bron van spiritualiteit* (Has an old hunger reeturned? Beauty as source of spirituality), Nijmegen: Valkhof, 2000; G. Danneels, *Christenen: Meer, beter of anders* (Christians: More, better or different), Mechelen: Aartsbisdom Mechelen, 2001; Pope John Paul II, 'Encycliek Evangelium Vitae: on the value and inviolability of human life', *Een-twee-een, Kerkelijke Documentatie*, 23 (1995) no 5, 212-289: Published in English: Catholic Truth Society, London (1995); P.A. van Gennip (Ed.), *Zakelijkheid met ziel: De bijdrage van ethiek en spiritualiteit aan maatschappelijk ondernemen en aan integer leiderschap* (Business with soul: the contribution of ethics and spirituality to social entrepreneurship and to leadership with integrity),

The empirical research referred to will research this motivation in more detail, to the extent that it is present among a representative sample of people connected to St Radboud. At the same time, they indicate that the job is not done and in fact never can be done. But that not done may be understood here as: we are on the road in faith.

It is the kind of faith that is also depicted in the proverb inscribed on the tower of the St Lebuinus Church in Deventer: *Fide Deo, Vigilia, Consule, Fortis Age*. In the translation by the Deventer poet G. Lugard jr.:

Have faith in God the Lord,
Survey with vigilant eyes,
Look before you leap,
But love brave deeds

Budel: Damon, 2002; College van Bestuur, *Kiezen voor kwaliteit: Strategisch plan, hoofdlijnen van strategisch beleid 2001-2005* (Choosing for quality: Strategic plan, main outline of strategic policy), Nijmegen: Catholic University, 2001; E.J.J.M. Kimman, *Goed verzorgd: Een handreiking voor medewerkers van het Catharina Ziekenhuis Eindhoven* (Well cared for: A helping hand for employees of the Catharina Hospital Eindhoven), 1993; H. Klamer & H. Pieper (Eds.), *Spiritualiteit in managen en besturen, een vruchtbare verbinding?* (Spirituality in management and administration: A fruitful connection?), Budel: Damon, 2003; J. Wessel-Ganzevoort, *Spiritualiteit in leiderschap* (Spirituality in leadership), Nijmegen: Valkhof Pers, 2003; Vereniging CVZKVZ, *Scholingsaanbod Zin en Zorg 2003* (Education provision Sense and Care), Gouda, 2002. Also see: M. Pijnenburg, 'Zin en zorg: Nieuw project van KVZ over de zin in de zorg' (Sense in care: New project by KVZ about sense in care), in: *Zin in zorg* (Sense in Care) 4 (2002) no 4, 22.

RESEARCH

H. JOCHEMSEN, M. KLAASE-CARPENTIER, B.S. CUSVELLER, A. VAN DE SCHEUR,
J. BOUWER

QUESTIONS OF LIFE AND DEATH IN THE TERMINAL PHASE TOWARDS QUALITY CRITERIA FOR SPIRITUAL CARE IN THE TERMINAL PALLIATIVE CARE FROM THE PATIENT'S PERSPECTIVE[1]

1. Introduction

Unquestionably, palliative care for people in the final phase of life has nowadays gained its own character, along with a new urgency. Recent decades have seen a great increase in the diagnostic and therapeutic possibilities of medicine. The powerful emphasis laid on health and life extension in our society has contributed to the fact that these medical options are also frequently applied to the last phase of life.

A moment arrives, however, where it has to be recognised that curing the patient is no longer practicable. The patient still has a considerable period to live, a period in which all sorts of complications and symptoms may occur that require specific care, including medical care. It is increasingly realised that care primarily directed to the treatment of symptoms in incurably ill patients, requires specific expertise, namely palliative (terminal) care. Palliative care for the patient in the terminal and pre-terminal phase of life contains all that is necessary to alleviate the patient's suffering and optimise his quality of life during its final period.[2]

[1] This contribution is based on the results of a study financed by ZonMw (Zorgonderzoek Nederland en Medische Wetenschappen van de Nederlandse Organisatie voor Wetenschappelijk Onderzoek (NOW) = Care research the Netherlands and Medical Science of the Netherlands Organisation for Academic Research). It is in principle applicable to every philosophy of life. The complete research report is published in: H. Jochemsen, M. Klaasse-Carpentier, B.S. Cusveller, G.G. van de Scheur & J. Bouwer, *Life questions in the terminal phase: Quality of spiritual care in the terminal palliative care from patient perspective*, Ede 2002 (Report from the Prof. dr. G.A.Lindenboom Instituut nr. 16). An adaptation from the point of view of Protestant Christian faith and directed to that population is in preparation.

[2] For a more detailed analysis of ethical and conceptual aspects of palliative care, see: R. Janssens & T. Quartier, 'Ethische und Konzeptionelle Aspekte der Palliativ Medizin', in: *Zeitschrift für Medizinische Ethik* 46 (2000), 273-286.

Speaking at as fundamental a level as possible, terminal care is caring and guiding people during their final phase of life. The way we attempt this is related to a view of being human. What place does dying have in this, or perhaps better put, what place does being human have in dying? Which aspects of being human belong to care during the phase of dying? It is not unusual in this connection to distinguish between the physical, psychological, social and spiritual aspects of being human *and* of care. In this connection we can refer to the WHO definition of palliative care.[3] This definition from an international institution of repute specifies spiritual problems, in addition to the psychological. In itself, this would seem sufficient reason to take these spiritual problems seriously as a special type of problem.

A few questions do then come up. What kind of problems should we think of here? And how may they be examined and to what quality demands should helpers responding to such problems meet? We have attempted to give answers to these questions in the research project we conducted. Four steps were established in broad lines here. These are, briefly formulated: (1) Define spirituality, and spiritual care; (2) Formulate a model for spirituality or choose a model for spirituality and adjust this if necessary to the Dutch situation; (3) Identify spiritual needs and requirements in terminal and pre-terminal patients; (4) Formulate guidelines for providing spiritual care and criteria for evaluating it.

We will work out these steps further in this contribution.

2. *Spirituality*

We approached the concept of spirituality from two points of view, namely from practice and from philosophy.

The practice, first of all. This is an approach stemming from the experience of deficiency. Care providers are in general very acquainted with somatic, social and psychological problems, everyone can name them. But at the same time they experience other sorts of problems that cannot be categorised under these headings. These are problems concerning interpretation of life and what happens to people, for example illness, suffering and death. They are termed existential problems or life problems. Yet we would like to speak about spiritual problems in this connection. Thus the interpretation of life, the meaning of life and of so-called 'life

[3] This definition is: 'Palliative care is the active total care for patients in the terminal phase of their life in which the incurable illness they suffer from no longer reacts to curative treatments and in which combating pain and other symptoms as well as dealing with social, psychological and spiritual problems should be paramount', see: *Tijdschrift voor Geneeskunde en Ethiek* (Journal for Medicine and Ethics) 9 (1999) no 4, supplement p. 1. This definition may to a certain extent be seen as a correction of the definition of health in which the spiritual dimension is not mentioned.

events' then has to do with spirituality. This approach deriving from the experience of care providers generally arouses recognition. Spiritual problems can be mentioned in this way, without care providers feeling that this applies to something that does not concern them or is very abstract.

The second approach is from philosophy, in particular the philosophical anthropology. From this point of departure too, it can be observed that man is in active relationship to his life and to his experiences. He interprets and comes to terms with this from a whole universe of symbols, motives and opinions, whether systematically ordered or not. It applies to all people, and not only to subscribers to an organised religion, that they are involved in what they perceive as 'essential and fundamental' in existence, and that they allow for this in organising their lives.[4] What people see as essential and fundamental, in other words as 'determining reality',[5] may have bearing on a higher spiritual Power, but also on matters such as happiness, or humanity for example. This involvement in the reality deemed as determining, also manifests itself in a religion and/or philosophy of life.[6] We understand by religion here, an organised religion, both in its form and its content. We understand by philosophy of life the entirety of beliefs, conscious or not, made about what is essential and fundamental in human existence and in our world, and along with this its meaning.[7] *We mean by spirituality in this research, the philosophy of life and religious functioning of man in the above-mentioned sense,*

4 Also see: 'Spirituality may be viewed as the actions and interactions of an embodied human actor who is facing death and creating a personally meaningful social world, a constructed world that can be either a resource or an encumbrance' (Daaleman & VandeCreek, 'Placing religions and spirituality in end-of-life care', in: *JAMA* 284 (2000) no 19, 2516). Although spirituality does not limit itself to situations in which the human being is face to face with death (unless one sees this as characteristic for the whole of human existence) and we approach it more in a phenomenological and constructivist way, this description contains important elements for the context of this study.

5 This also comes to the fore in the last description of the concept of religions given by *Webster's Third New International Dictionary*. This description is as follows: '7a: A cause, principle, system of tenets held with ardor, devotion, conscientiousness, and faith: a value held to be of supreme importance. b: a quality, condition, custom, or thing, inspiring zealous devotion, conscientious maintenance, and cherishing'; for the term 'religious' this dictionary gives the following illustration: '1: relating to that which is acknowledged as ultimate reality: manifesting devotion to and reflecting the nature of the divine or that which one holds to be of ultimate importance'. Here too religiosity viewed as a general human characteristic, in other words, as an anthropological structure.

6 According to M. van den Berg, *Zingeving in de palliatieve zorg* (Meaning in palliative care), Houten: Bohn Stafleu Van Loghum, 2001, 11, which also counts faith, religion and philosophy of life to the spiritual area.

7 Acc. the definition of philosophy of life by Van Willigenburg et al. in: T. van Willigenburg et al., *Ethiek, levensbeschouwing en het management in instellingen voor intramurale gezondheidszorg* (Ethics, philosophy of life and the management in institutions for intramural healthcare), Utrecht: Nationaal Ziekenhuisinstituut, 1991, 20.

to which the questions of experiencing of meaning and the giving of meaning must also thus be ascribed. And as religiosity always manifests itself in an actual human life in a *particular* belief and in a *particular* philosophy of life and possibly a *particular* religion, so too spirituality obtains *particular* form and content in an actual human life derived from out of the philosophy and/or religion adhering to it. In this research, we have been almost solely concerned with spirituality in the same anthropological and functional sense with which we discussed religiosity above. What does this signify for the concept of spirituality?

It means that spirituality is seen as a way of existence for all people and not only for people adhering to a particular religion in the sense of a organized religion. Although it is likewise clear that a religion, but also a philosophy of life not based on religion, plays a particular role in their spirituality for its adherents. It further signifies that spirituality is not a *separate domain* of human existence (for example the participation in specific rituals at specific times), but is an *aspect* of the *wholeness* of existence. Thus it is an *attitude to life* rather than a *sphere in life.* Although a specific sphere in life, keeping certain religious customs for example, can occupy a very important place in forming and nourishing that attitude to life.

Regardless of our own Protestant Christian belief, we have chosen this functional approach here. This is in view of society's pluralistic character and the fact that spirituality is always present in every care practice, regardless of the specific interpretation that people give to it. For ideologically determined images, motivations, experiences and beliefs on life and illness, suffering, death, the meaning of care, etc. always partly play a role in care in some kind of way. That practice is in itself not only normatively but also spiritually charged. Spirituality is not something that is added like icing on the cake to a technically defined professional practice. Spirituality is always there already, whether or not people realise this or not. If one does not realise this, then one presumably has a completely technical and functional idea of practice and the pursuance of that practice will be characterised by that 'spirituality'. One fears that this happens on occasion. Philosophies of life and religion have been forced into the private domain to a significant degree in our society. There is also often an attitude prevalent in care, and particularly in the medical occupational group: this is a profession – and that is then understood relatively technically – and the rest is private. As if faith and the 'facts of medicine' are two separate worlds. Countless choices in care provision, also in medical care, are made on the basis of normative considerations that are related to beliefs about life, health, illness and suffering and their significance. A particular spirituality is always expressed in every actual care practice.[8] Thus the provision of care always implicitly includes a form

---

[8] See also H. Jochemsen & G. Glas, *Verantwoord medisch handelen: Naar een proeve van een christelijke medische ethiek* (Responsible medical care, towards a Christian medical ethics), Amsterdam: Buijten & Schipperheijn, 1997, esp. ch.3 and 4.

of 'spiritual care' in the sense of a complying – explicitly or not – with the spiritual functioning of the care seeker. It is therefore desirable that every caregiver should contemplate that aspect of his or her care provision and ask what is its significance for him or herself and those seeking care. Integral care also implies that the needs and requirements of the patient in the spiritual sphere are also examined and that they are met as well as possible. Although many caregivers in the pursuance of their practice may well give more attention to this spiritual dimension than their own explicit views on practice might lead one to surmise.

3. Model for spirituality

Now we have determined that a form of spiritual care belongs to integral care provision, the question arises as to how spirituality may be put into practice. The concept itself is too broad to be able to derive a tangible care provision from it.

In the literature we found, in our view, a practicable division of spirituality into themes by the American spiritual carer and researcher George Fitchett and co-workers.[9] Instead of pastoral diagnostics we should speak of spiritual diagnostics.

a. The model assumes a holistic approach to spirituality in the sense that spirituality is closely linked to other dimensions of human existence;
b. The model assumes a functional approach to spirituality in the sense that spirituality is seen as an anthropological structure;
c. The model has an extensive empirical basis, so that it is not necessary to provide exhaustive empirical material as support for the model.

The model is briefly reproduced in table 1.

TABLE 1 FITCHETT'S 7X7 MODEL FOR PASTORAL DIAGNOSTICS

Holistic dimensions	*Spiritual dimensions*
medical	faith and significance
psychological	calling and consequences
family system	experience and emotions
psycho-social	courage and growth
ethnic and cultural	rituals and practices
social	living in community
spiritual	authority and leadership

9 G. Fitchett, *Assessing spiritual needs: A guide for caregivers*, Augsburg: Fortress, 1993; see also J. Bouwer, *Pastorale diagnostiek: Modellen en mogelijkheden* (Pastoral diagnostics: Models and opportunities), Zoetermeer: Boekencentrum, 1998.

From this model, we have only used the division into themes belonging to the spiritual dimension

A small scale research among care providers in terminal palliative care taught us that this model may be recognised in the situation to which we primarily address ourselves, but that a few terminological adaptations were desirable. Suggestions for adaptation were given. We have incorporated these. In addition, later analysis of interviews with terminal and pre-terminal patients and of the literature has led to a few further terminological adaptations. The thematic division we used to further develop the quality instruments intended, is in table 2. Further details of the concept of spirituality are here elaborated in themes and sub-themes, so that it more approaches the actual provision of care. We have illustrated the themes after making two preliminary remarks. Firstly, that this summing up is not to say that all these themes and sub-themes must explicitly come up for everyone. They are themes that may play a role and will be variously operant between one person and the next.

Our second note is that we do not discuss this material in the interview in the same manner as the spiritual carer would do so. This will depend among other things on the personal philosophy of life of the spiritual carer and on the setting.

Faith, philosophy of life and meaning

The first theme is faith, philosophy of life and meaning. These concepts are here intended in the narrower sense of the content of someone's faith or ideology. Every creed and religious community has to a certain extent a language, symbols of its own, and its own way of creating meaning. Although deriving from the functional approach of spirituality, the latter is formulated in a more constructivist way, than we undertstand our faith at any rate. At its most profound the Christian faith, but in our opinion also faith in other religions and philosophies of life, is founded upon a form of revelation, even although the origin of that revelation will differ. This does not alter the fact that there is always an element of human processing in specific convictions and the experiencing of faith, and in the interpretation of symbols. The relationship of this theme to the situation of diseases that are sometimes terminal, thus leads to sub-themes of the significance of illness and suffering to the meaning of life, in the way this meaning is interpreted by those involved.

TABLE 2 THEMATICISING SPIRITUALITY ACCORDING TO ADAPTED MODEL OF FITCHETT *CUM SUIS*

Theme	*Explanation*
1 Faith, philosophy of life, meaning	Conviction Symbolic significance of objects/language Way in which meaning is created Significance of illness/suffering for the meaningof life
2 Goal in life, life balance	Expression of spiritual dimension Consequences of illness for faith/philosophy of life Naming of illness in relationship to society/work/life task Ethical principles for behaviour What has been the direction of life? Has life been what one had imagined?
3 Experiences and emotions	Religious experiences Emotions linked to religious experiences Emotions linked to coming to terms with illness
4 Courage, hope, growth	Sources of power that give/gave the courage to keep going in difficult circumstances Experiences of personal growth and re-orientation through the crisis
5 Rituals and customs	Which form a part of the life history and which are still important? Influence of situation or illness on rituals and customs and the experiencing of them
6 Relationships and social connections	Community of rituals and convictions Support from community in coming to terms Help and care providers Support in coming to terms Treatment of care providers Communication/use of language Care for continuity Openness in talking to others about situation or illness Influence of illness on relationships and solidarity with others Reconciliation and restoration of relationships

7 Orientation and guiding principles	From whom is approval sought for personal convictions, faith, rituals/uses? Relationship between ideas on philosophy of life and medical/nursing treatment Who/what is exemplary function/source of inspiration

Goal and balance in life

This is something that many people chiefly deal with in the final phase of life. A human being looks back once again in this final phase of life and asks himself: What have I actually done with my life? Sometimes it is difficult for people to put this into words. In the first instance it might be something on a very practical level. A good craftsman or woman in one field or another. Wanting to be a good father, a good mother for the children. Such matters may have been connected in some way to a personal spirituality and to the experiencing of meaning to an important degree. There can be a lot of disappointment in the opportunities life has offered one or in the opportunities that one has availed oneself of. A question in the final phase of life not only concerns how you yourself feel you have done, there is also the question of experience of meaning if you are no longer able to work on a personal 'life project'. Who are you in your own eyes if you can no longer do anything? What does that signify for the experience of spirituality? Do you then still feel accepted and valued?

Experiences and emotions

Here experiences and emotions described as facets of the grief process by Kübler Ross for example, may also play a role. Yet not merely these and not even in a predominant place. These are primarily concerned with psychological functioning. Here we are chiefly concerned with the experience and emotions directly connected with philosophy of life, faith and religion. A very clear example is a conversion experience or another religious or spiritual experience. Such experiences, or the lack of them, may play a very great role in certain faith traditions. Sometimes conversion is seen as something that must be accompanied by an exceptional experience, sometimes worked out in specific steps, if it is to be considered real. If such an experience is lacking, then it is questionable whether one is a real believer. Other examples in this connection are experiences of the clear presence of God or being forsaken by God on the other hand, or an experience of an existential loneliness. And it is therefore very important that such experiences and their significance can be discussed with understanding. As an aside, it should be noted here that these examples do make it clear that in the experience of the care seeker, spiritual care and pastoral care in particular may best be given by someone who shares the religious convictions of the care seeker.

Courage, hope and growth

What sources of strength which give or have given courage in difficult circumstances does one draw upon? Where does one get the strength from to keep on going? It is marvellous how people in the final phase sometimes seem to have sources of strength that they themselves were not even aware of, but that suddenly bear fruit again. And a facet of guidance is helping to seek the sources of strength, by which people live. This does not mean to say that other things may not be offered, but it is certainly important to trace where and how people are. A subtheme here is that people – in the critical confrontation with their own death – experience personal growth, orientate themselves anew, and that their relationships may deepen. It does happen that the final period of life may well be experienced as the most valuable one of allbecause of this. But this too cannot be generalised.

Rituals and customs

Which spiritual (religious) customs and practices form a part of someone's life and life story? Which still continue to do so? Within the Christian tradition one may think of baptism. Although occurring a while ago it may play an important role in the experience of religion. Further, Communion/the Eucharist, but also prayer and intercession. People within other traditions naturally have other important matters. It is a good thing for care providers to get to know these. One problem is that being ill can sometimes hinder participation in such activities. What can an institution do to meet people's needs as much as possible regarding the rituals and customs essential to a care seeker?

Relationships and social bonds

To which community, family, residential community, group, does the person belong? The support of the community in coming to terms with being incurably ill is very important. Man is also a social being. Care providers can be sometimes so focussed on their task of providing care that they lose sight of the fact that very essential contributions in this area might also be made by the immediate family and friends. The personal network and volunteer help, as it is also called.

Yet the help of caregivers belongs here too. For a striking finding of our research into terminal and pre-terminal patients was that the possibility of experiencing meaning in the terminal phase is also influenced to an important extent by the quality of relationships, including those with caregivers. If these relationships are bad, if people feel that they are actually too much for a caregiver or for a certain care setting, then the eventuality of meaningful experience becomes much more difficult. The 'everyday' quality of care may have great repercussions for spiritual experience and the openness of the care seeker to spiritual care. Treatment is very important here, likewise communication, care for continuity, openness to discussing the condition of the disease with others. Sometimes people scarcely dare to speak of their (incurable) illness for fear that people will find that unpleasant and then no longer visit. They then have to process everything on their own, unless that pattern is broken.

Reconciliation, restoration of relationships befits this theme too. Settling quarrels, strengthening loosened ties to family members. Extending and receiving forgiveness from people and, for those for whom this is a possibility, finding forgiveness from God. Very crucial topics for which spiritual care may fulfil a supportive and guiding role are also familiar subject matter of course.

Orientation and guidelines

This involves the question as to who is seen as source or reference point for a philosophy of life and faith and normative convictions. In other words, whose approval is judged of value regarding personal conviction and faith. This may be an authority, this may be a book, for example the Bible. But it may also be persons. The relationship between ideological conviction and the norms one wishes to abide by in medical and nursing treatment also play a role here. To proceed or not with a treatment in a final phase of life. People also often look for support for such decisions. In their own philosophy or in other people, for example a minister in the religious community to which they belong. In some Jewish communities a Rabbi has exceptional authority, even in these kinds of decisions.

4. From spiritual needs and requirements to criteria

The third step in our research is to identify the spiritual needs and requirements of people who are receiving terminal palliative care, based on open interviews with questions inspired by the themes of the Fitchett model, and based on literature. The texts of open interviews are analysed in an extensive qualitative process. Starting point was the question of which problems, desires and requirements does the pre-terminal and terminal patient experience in the sphere of spirituality.

This analysis led to a list of needs, requirements and desires in this sphere, that were subsequently ordered according to the Fitchett model; some new adjustments were then made to that model. A similar analysis of requirements and desires regarding spirituality was carried out into literature on spiritual care in the terminal phase of life. The results of both analysis were subsequently integrated into a overview of such requirements and desires of people receiving palliative care in the final phase of life, ordered according to the modified Fitchett model.

In the following step, step 4, activities were derived from those formulations of needs, requirements and desires which might accommodate them.[10] Those activities in their turn are formulated in a functional way, thus without interpretation of spiritual care as regards content. The result of the whole analysis is a list of care transactions including the attitude required to meet the full breadth of the patient needs, requirements and desires we identified in the sphere of spiritual care. This list can therefore function as a list of criteria for the quality of such care.[11]

These criteria are ordered according to the modified Fitchett model. We added an 0-theme to the themes named in it. That involves somatic care and all sorts of preconditions for good care. Our research indicated that as a rule spiritual care only comes into its own if certain quality criteria are met for care in general. Further a distinction is made per theme between the level of organisation and of individual assistance. Direct spiritual care occurs through individual assistance, but certain criteria should also be met at organisation level and the preconditions, in order to arrive at good spiritual care. Thus the criteria for the organisation primarily concern management and leadership, those on the care level concern the caregivers. In addition, the caregivers' list has been reformulated as a questionnaire assessing patient satisfaction with the spiritual care offered, in other words quality of care from the patient perspective. The question of who provides the care designated in the diverse criteria, is also relevant when providing spiritual care to the individual care seeker. We have consciously refused to spread the diverse criteria over professional groups because in our view such a general spread is not possible. We would like, however, to make a few remarks on this point.

a. Spiritual carers may be expected to be able to provide spiritual care over the whole breadth of the criteria and with the required depth.
b. This cannot be expected of other caregivers, but they should be able to a least spot care seeker's questions and requirements in this sphere and refer

10 See Jochemsen et al., *Life questions in the terminal phase*, esp. ch. 4.

11 Quality as the degree to which the justified expectations of the user are met. The limitation 'justified' does not so much concern the care seeker as the caregiver whose care giving must fit within the professional context and must be compatible with his conscience. Not everyone from his own faith will, for example, be able to actively participate with certain religious customs and will not be able to honour any desires that care seekers might have had in this area.

them adequately to a spiritual carer or another person that the care seeker wishes to consult, for example a clergyman of his own community.[12]

c. Certain caregivers in a palliative team, for example nurses, could specialise further. They would later be equipped to provide much more far reaching spiritual care than might be expected of the average fellow professional. The precise division of tasks will therefore depend on the situation and the composition of the team.

5. *Testing in practice*

The criteria we obtained through the above-mentioned process were presented to diverse groups of care providers and patients (representatives) to be judged on completeness, intelligibility and usability. They were asked to score each criterion on 'very important', 'important' or 'not important', and to give an open commentary. Seventy two completed lists were returned from managers, spiritual carers, caregivers and volunteers/patient association representatives.[13] Processing the commentary we got in our provisional lists of key points and criteria, which eventually led to the final lists included as appendices after this chapter (appendix 1 and 2).

These lists have been presented anew to care providers, namely some general practitioners and care providers in hospices, palliative care units in hospitals, nursing homes and care homes. They were asked to use the lists for some time or to go through them carefully from the point of view of their own practice experience (general practitioners do not usually have a variety of cases of death within a few months). They were also asked to comment on them for reliability, form, length, use of language, information and suchlike. The commentary obtained was incorporated in reviewing and reformulating the lists of key points and the list of criteria for specifying patient satisfaction. This version is published by the Prof. Dr. G.A. Lindeboom Institute in a convenient form.

---

[12] Cf. R.R van Leeuwen & B.S. Cusveller, *Verpleegkundig competentieprofiel zorg voor spiritualiteit* (Nursing competence profile care for spirituality), Ede 2002 (Report from the Prof. dr. G.A. Lindeboom Institute, nr. 17).

[13] For the details see Jochemsen et al., *Life questions in the terminal phase*, ch.5. The response is quantitatively difficult to indicate in that some people made copies of the lists, that were subsequently completed by colleagues, and this is not so important in this qualitative research. Globally, it can be said that most criteria were considered very important or important and that we have scrapped criteria that were not considered important. Further suggestions to do with formulation have been incorporated as well as possible.

Appendix 1

SPIRITUAL CARE IN THE TERMINAL PHASE OF LIFE

Policy for board, middle management, spiritual carers, doctors, nurses and carers

Prof. dr. G.A. Lindeboom Institute

THEME 0. CONDITIONS FOR PROVIDING SPIRITUAL CARE

A. Points of attention for the assistor

Attitude

- The assistor shows involvement, empathy and respect for behaviour, philosophy of life, wishes and feelings of the care seeker
- The assistor can cope with his own feelings and guards his own boundaries.
- The assistor respects the confidential relationship with the care seeker (confidentiality).
- The assistor recognises and discusses any mistakes with the care seeker.

Care process

- The assistor pays careful attention to the need to combat pain and symptoms, physical care and nutrition of the care seeker.
- Appointments with the care seeker are recorded and kept.
- The assistor takes care for the continuity of care during transferral of the care seeker from home to the institution or vice versa.

Information and permission

- The assistor gives the care seeker (preferably with a second listener) clear information on the illness, course of the illness, treatment options and the pros- and cons of this.
- The assistor informs the care seeker about the possibilities and limits of care at home or in an institution.
- The assistor gives the care seeker time to consider permission for examination, treatment (curative or palliative) and/or admittance to hospital.

B. Points of attention for the organisation

Personnel

- The organisation promotes an attitude of the personnel like the one stated above and gives guidance for this or supervision
- The organisation has specialist assistors who can offer palliative care.
- The organisation offers the care seeker the possibility of daily contact with a spiritual carer.
- The organisation can quickly anticipate care seekers' wishes.

Services

- The organisation has a description of the different disciplines with their responsibilities
- The organisation has a system for calling in other specialists
- The organisation has information material on the illness and illness process, and on the pros and cons of examination and treatment.

- The organisation has a system of recording appointments with care seekers.
- The organisation has a space where conversations may be carried out with the care seeker and his family/those close to him.
- The organisation has an arrangement (confidential person, complaints commission) for the dealing with mistakes and complaints.

THEME 1. FAITH AND PHILOSOPHY OF LIFE

A. Points of attention for the assistor

Significance
- The assistor helps the care seeker, if desired, to investigate what the philosophy of life, aim and meaning of his life, and is illness and death mean to him.

Guidance
- The assistor attempts to acknowledge, discuss and support the process of assimilation of the care seeker.

B. Points of attention for the organisation

Personnel
- The organisation has specialist personnel that supports the care seeker in the process of assimilating being sick in the light of his philosophy of life.

Service
- The organisation has a service to, in consultation with the care seeker, to establish information about his philosophy of life, and any religious customs.

THEME 2. LIFE AIM AND LIFE BALANCE

A. Points of attention for the assistor

Taking stock
- The assistor observes and discusses any needs of the care seeker and his friends and family to look back and forward at life.

Experiencing loss
- The assistor supports the care seeker and his friends and family if desired, in experiencing loss or change in his life circumstances(for example, private life, family, work, other activities).

Rounding off
- The assistor helps to record which responsibilities and tasks the care seeker sees for himself and supports him in realising wishes in this area.
- The assistor calls in a specialist at the request of the care seeker to look after his material affairs.

THEME 3. EXPERIENCES AND EMOTIONS

A. Points of attention for assistor

Dealing with emotions

- The assistor knows how to recognises need in the case of a wish for death possibly expressed by the care seeker and discusses the policy of his general practitioner or of the institution.
- The assistor shows understanding for the care seeker who clings to life and tries to help him to express this, to comfort and to guide him.
- The assistor can observe the care seeker's need to make spiritual pain discussable and tries, at his request, to help him deal with it.
- The assistor shows understanding for and tries to support the care seeker processing loss of physical and psychological functions.
- The assistor can observe psychological defence mechanisms and deal with them.

Referral

- The assistor consults if necessary other specialists regarding assimilation processess (for example psychologist, music therapist, spiritual carer).

B. Points of attention for the organisation

Personnel

- The organisation has specialist personnel that realises the emotional significance of dying and that can support the care seeker in the process of assimilation.
- The organisation offers opportunities for supervision or coaching of personnel regarding emotional expressions about death.

Service

- The organisation has policy for dealing with a wish for death and takes care that this is known on admission.

THEME 4. COURAGE, HOPE AND GROWTH

A. Points of attention for the assistor

- The assistor attempts to help the care seeker to penetrate sources if possible (such as faith and philosophy of life) from which he can draw hope, courage and strength.
- The assistor observes changes in the care seeker's self image and can make this discussable if need be.

B. Points of attention for the organisation

- The organisation offers opportunities for the care seeker to find access to sources from which the care seeker can draw strength.

THEME 5. RELIGIOUS CUSTOMS AND PRACTICE

A. Points of attention for the assistor

Support
- The assistor informs the care seeker about religious activities in the organisation.
- The assistor discusses which religious customs and/or practices are important to the care seeker and his friends and family and tries to support participation in them.
- The assistor investigates which specific customs and practices are important to the care seeker and his friends and family around the departure of the care seeker.

Definition of expertise
- The assistor can indicate his own boundaries when the care seeker requests him to participate in religious practices.
- The assistor calls in, at the request of the care seeker, the help of a spiritual carer.

B. Points of attention for the organisation

Personnel
- The organisation has personnel that has knowledge of and respect for cultural differences and religious expression.

Services
- The planning of care is geared to the religious activities of the care seeker.
- The organisation has a space for meditation-, quiet and meeting.

THEME 6. RELATIONSHIPS AND SOCIAL TIES

A. Points of attention for the assistor

Attention to contacts
- The assistor asks the care seeker on admittance (and notes it down) which relationships are or were important to him.
- The assistor asks the care seeker on admittance whether a religious community or church is important and contacts this at the request of the care seeker.
- The assistor attempts to help the care seeker, if desired, to improve the quality of relationships with friends and family (make meeting possible, supporting reconcilliation, making communication blocks discussable).

Attention to friends and family
- The assistor informs the care seeker about the possibilities of accommodation that the organisation offers to his friends and family.
- The assistor supports the care seeker and his friends and family in the case of the approaching departure.
- The assistor offers supervision to the friends and family of the deceased in connection with the mourning process.

B. Points of attention for the organisation

Personnel

- The organisation offers opportunities for supervision of coaching of the personnel regarding the process of assimilation and supervision of care seekers and their social network.

Service

- The organisation offers as flexible a visiting arrangement possible for the care seeker.
- The organisation has possibilities of accommodation and means of communication for friends and family.

THEME 7. ORIENTATION SOURCE AND GUIDELINES

A. Points of attention for the assistor

Autonomy van the care seeker

- The assistor recognises that dying is a process that the care seeker undergoes himself and at the same time touches all those around.
- The assistor supports the care seeker, if desired, in taking his own decisions.
- The assistor discusses who can advise the care seeker, if desired, in the case of ethical decisions around setting up, continuing and ceasing treatment (for example, drip feeding, infusion).

Appendix 2

SPIRITUAL CARE IN THE TERMINAL PHASE OF LIFE
Evaluation form for patients or their representatives

Clarification
This evaluation form contains the most central points of attention from the assistance for the quality of spiritual care in the terminal phase. It is used in combination with the assistance for assistors and/or the policy for the organisation. This form is intended to determine the response of patients and/or their representatives to the spiritual care provided and to adjust the quality. Spiritual care is an inseparable part of total care. Even more, if the other parts of care- somatic, psychological and social – obtain sufficient attention, then there is space for the spiritual, which was apparent from interviews with terminally ill patients. Theme 0 indicates the basal points of attentions for care that according to terminal patients are an absolute condition for good spiritual care.

Please complete the circle that best reflects your answer.
Y = Yes, N = No, NA = Not applicable

General quality criteria of care as condition for spiritual care

	Y	N	NA
1. I am satisfied about the involvement of the assistors.	O	O	O
2. I am satisfied about my care.	O	O	O
3. I was carefully informed about my illness and my treatment possibilities	O	O	O
4. I had sufficient opportunity and support for taking decisions myself aboutcare and treatment.	O	O	O

1. Faith and philosophy of life

1. I experience sufficient space and respect for my faith or philosophy of life.	O	O	O
2. I experience sufficient space and support for my questions on the aim and the meaning of my life and of my illness.	O	O	O

2. Aim in life and taking stock

1. I experience sufficient space and respect while looking back on my life and to the future.	O	O	O
2. I experience sufficient space and respect while completing my responsibilities and tasks in my life.	O	O	O

3. Experiences and emotions

1. I experience sufficient understanding for my desire not to have to live any more	O	O	O
2. I experience sufficient understanding for my need to cling to life.	O	O	O
3. I experience sufficient space and respect for my emotions around my approaching departure.	O	O	O

4. Courage, hope and growth

1. I experience sufficient help in finding sources that give me strength to keep on living. O O O
2. I experience sufficient support in learning to cope with the changes in my life. O O O

5. Religious customs and practices

1. I am informed about church services, remembrance services and other gatherings in the institution to my satisfaction. O O O
2. I experience sufficient time and respect for my religious activities. O O O
3. I am brought into contact with a spiritual carer of my choice to my satisfaction. O O O

6. Relationships

1. I have sufficient opportunity to have contact with my religious community or church. O O O
2. I have sufficient opportunity to meet my family, friends, neighbours and colleagues. O O O
3. We are sufficiently informed about the support and accommodation possibilities for my friends and family. O O O

7. Orientation source and guidelines

1. I have sufficient support in taking ethical decisions about my care and treatment. O O O

K.E. Bras

MEDITATION AS SPIRITUAL INTERVENTION FOR THE PSYCHOSOCIAL GUIDANCE OF PEOPLE WITH CANCER

I consider meditation a spiritual discipline. This enables me to make a connection between spirituality and meditation. There is much discussion about what spirituality is. Among other things, this involves the plurality of our culture, where the form and content of spirituality in various sub cultures are increasingly diverse in nature. Because I have done research into meditation within centres open to people with very different philosophy of life backgrounds, I seek an interpretation of the concept of spirituality which is recognisable to as many people as possible. I therefore agree with Aalders' definition: 'Wherever man is engaged in making his life comply with a *transcendent* giving of meaning, with conscious intention and in a more or less methodical manner, there is spirituality'.[1] Aalders' italics emphasise the concept *transcendent*, meaning the self transcendence of man here, enabling him to rise above his own limitations, transcending his own sphere. He considers this endeavour of man to be an anthropological constant, which may be interpreted both religiously and a-religiously. Transcending a personal sphere signifies more here than the increasing of possibilities for action. It has primarily to do with a contemplative openness to the inexhaustible secret of reality. Aalders speaks here of reality as 'bearer of a deep secret; of a hidden and yet audible Meaning, an intriguing Order, often even an observable Word'.[2]

Spiritual disciplines are needed to organise life and shape it around this transcendence. Aalders mentions meditation in addition to asceticism. He sees meditation as a means of calling the disorganised and uncontrolled life of the mind 'to order'. The mind can open itself to the true nature of reality through the discipline of inner and outer stillness that one submits oneself to.

---

1 C. Aalders, *Spiritualiteit: Geestelijk leven vroeger en nu* (Spirituality: Spiritual life past and present), 's Gravenhage 1980 (3th ed.; Praktisch Theologische Handboekjes 31), 13.

2 Aalders, *Spiritualiteit*, 23

In association with Aalders's ideas, I perceive meditation as a spiritual discipline, a consciously and methodically applied means to make life increasingly fulfil a sense of transcendence. Meditation, however, is also used as an intervention in the psychosocial counselling of people with physical and/or psychological symptoms. The questions is, in how far and in what way may meditation still be considered a spiritual discipline? In other words, what relationship then exists between this meditative intervention and spirituality? The aim of my research is to explore this question.

In this article, I will report on a research into the use of meditation in the counselling of people with cancer in three centres in the Netherlands, and will report on an attention training based on *vipassana* meditation that I myself took part in. Prior to this, I will make a brief summary of a literature research into the significance of meditation for people with psychological and/or physical symptoms, which I hope to publish elsewhere. The names of the participants in meditation interviewed are fictitious for reasons of privacy.

The literature research

Much literature has been published on the significance that meditation may have for people with psychological and/or physical symptoms. What people understand by meditation is important here. I myself use a definition covering as many kinds of meditation as possible:

> Meditation is the cultivation of a mental attitude that, no longer determined by cognitive and attitudinal stereotypes from everyday life, is open to the inner and outer reality in its 'being so' and for its participation in being transcendent.

Distinction is made between an active mental attitude and a more receptive one on occasion. In the latter mode of consciousness, we are released from the stereotypes with which we safeguard ourselves in daily life and utilise to satisfy our needs. When one is freed from this attitude of mind engraved with prejudices and interests, one is more open to inner and outer reality such as it really is. One then also experiences in this being so of the inner and outer world a profundity that one calls transcendence. That is to say, the deeper significance of reality has withdrawn from reasoning intellect, but may be experienced as a sort of total-experience. How this 'transcendence' is subsequently interpreted is dependent on the philosophy of life behind the way one lives.

In every religion meditation was traditionally and is still an important means of entering this receptive attitude of mind and experiencing the transcendent depth of reality. But in recent decades, meditation is also applied in therapeutic contexts such as pain control, stress reduction training, cognitive therapies, psychosocial counselling of people with serious illnesses, etc. Reference is made here to the physical and mental effects confirmed by research, such as muscular relaxation, lower blood pressure, calmer heartbeat, less use of oxygen, other brain waves, increased ability to control stress and depression. The more recent insights of psycho-immunology indicating that stress reduction through meditation is beneficial to the immune system are also referred to. Increasing patient awareness and independence has led to a large quantity of self-help techniques aiding active contribution to one's own health and wellbeing. Meditation techniques are included in this. A superabundance of research results demonstrates the therapeutic significance of a deep physical and mental relaxation, and meditative relaxation has in any case proved its usefulness.[3]

In addition, meditation has traditionally been focussed on acquiring another attitude to life and attitude of mind. Some forms of therapeutic meditation are also aimed at this. Patients accordingly learn that they are more than their symptoms, that in the depth of their being they form part of a greater entity. This can give them a sense of being profoundly 'whole', and the surrender to that 'wholeness' can help them to surrender with more faith to the here and now, with its opportunities and limitations. In this respect, spirituality is often referred to as a sense of inner connection to the 'great totality' or the 'transcendent being'. I should just like to consider these forms of meditation as spiritual intervention, that are not only aimed at relaxation or stress reduction, but also strive for a spiritual attitude of mind. In my research I have especially focussed on two forms of meditation, namely the 'attention training' or 'stress reduction training' as developed by Kabat-Zinn, and the Christian contemplative prayer utilised by Finney in his psychotherapy.[4]

Attention training (mindfulness meditation) developed out of the Buddhist *Vipasanna* meditation, but is offered in an ideologically neutral sense. Kabat-Zinn worked at a clinic for pain control at the University of Massachusetts and thousands of people with different physical symptoms have been treated in the programme developed there in the meantime. The research he published clearly

---

3 See for an extensive overview of the literature in this field M.G.T. Kwee (Ed.), *Psychotherapy, meditation & health: A cognitive-behavioural perspective*, London-The Hague 1990, 22-29.

4 Kabat-Zinn's attention training or stress reduction programme is expounded in J. Kabat-Zinn, *Handboek meditatief ontspannen: Effectief programma voor het bestrijden van pijn en stress* (Manual meditative relaxing: Effective programme for combating pain), Haarlem 2000. The use of contemplative prayer is expounded by Finney in an unpublished dissertation of which I have a photocopy: J.R. Finney, *Contemplative prayer as an adjunct to psychotherapy* (dissertation presented to the faculty of the Graduate School of Psychology, Fuller Theological Seminary, Pasadena 1984).

highlighted the positive effects of this programme. It was interesting that this programme also appeared to work in a psychotherapeutic context. A few cognitive therapists published a thorough research into this.[5] The attention training was deployed here within a cognitive therapy for people who had several depressions. The therapy was intended to prevent a new depression.

The psychologist John R. Finney did research into the effect of contemplative prayer on people undergoing psychotherapy. Although this concerned a limited research among a small group of patients, there are clear indications that this form of Christian meditation was considered a positive contribution to their therapy by those concerned.

Many questions remain, such as; which aspects in which form of meditation have the most effect? How can one distinguish between the effects of meditation and the uncontrolled effects of, for example, the group process? How can one make room in ideologically neutrally offered meditation for the participants' spiritual experiences and which unspoken spiritual assumptions of the meditation supervisors play an unchecked role? How does one prevent the relationship to God in religious forms of meditation being reduced to a therapeutic effect? It is striking that there is still almost no research done into the therapeutic effect of explicitly religious, including Christian, forms of meditation. The question as to the role of spirituality in meditation training and the therapeutic significance of this has scarcely been researched at all. It is specifically on this point that my experiences in three centres for psychosocial counselling of people with cancer may make a contribution.

My research in three centres for psychosocial counselling

The Helen Dowling Institute

The Helen Dowling Institute (HDI) is situated in Utrecht, The Netherlands. Prof. Dr. M.J. De Vries, a cell biologist who wished to do research into the effects of bio-psychological counselling, founded the HDI fifteen years ago. The objectives have broadened in the meantime and the Institute itself also offers counselling. Lastly, it also places its knowledge, skill and experience in the service of the advancement of others' expertise in the field of cancer. The research attempts to find answers to the question as to what relationship exists between medical and psychological factors playing a role in the origin and course of cancer. This counselling is aimed at the psychological and social problems accompanying cancer for

[5] Z.V. Segal, J.M.G. Williams & J.D. Teasdale, *Mindfulness-based cognitive therapy for depression: A new approach to preventing relapse*, New York-London 2002.

patients and their environment. The point of departure here is that people are *more* than their cancer alone. The approach is more 'person orientated' than 'tumour orientated'. No readymade solutions are offered and those offering assistance do not take over the wheel from the patient.

There are different forms of counselling. The counselling most suitable is selected at intake. That might be individual counselling, with or without the partner or with the family. In addition there are four forms of group counselling. There is a base group 'Working on coping' that meets six times. There is a 'companion group' where one shares experiences with fellow sufferers in twelve weekly sessions. There is a 'Partner in adversity' group which meets once a week for 12 weeks. Participants share their experiences with one another. There is a 'Partner apart' group, intended, as the name indicates, for patients' partners. This group meets four times. Finally there is the course 'Living in the vortex', in which relaxation and meditation are central. I am particularly interested in this course.[6]

Conversation with Welmet Hudig

Welmet Hudig is a theologian-therapist. She has worked as chaplain in the Sofia Children's Hospital (Rotterdam, The Netherlands), and later trained as a psychosynthesis guide. She has been leading the 'Living in the vortex' course for a number of years, along with others.

The course consists of eight mornings and one day. The work uses the Jon Kabat-Zinn model, as described in his book *Full catastrophe living*.

People signing on have an intake interview first. Afterwards they are admitted to a group containing a maximum of fifteen participants. The sessions have the following sections. After a short relaxation exercise people exchange experiences about the recent past. Afterwards, a meditation exercise takes place (for example relaxation, yoga, sitting or walking meditation, visualisations, etc.). This leads to discussion of the meditation and how it can be used at home. The participants are given CDs with meditation instructions requiring roughly three-quarters of an hour per day (six days per week). Further there is a distinction made between formal meditation (sitting down and applying oneself) and informal meditation (building in meditative principles into your daily round). The course costs 300 Euro. Various health insurers compensate it.

According to the research, virtually all participants benefit from the course and are able to better deal with their illness afterwards, communicate better about it, and they suffer less from stress.

---

6 I obtained this information from the leaflet *Information for patients* from the Helen Dowling Institute. See

Research
The HDI regularly does academic research into the effects of this counselling. The results of this research are published. The last research publication concerned 2000. I have taken the data below from this report.[7] An evaluation of the personal counselling was published in 1996. Now an evaluation of two group activities is offered: namely four groups of the 'Companion group' and three groups of the 'Living in the vortex' course. Three areas of attention are central in the evaluation:

1. What are the experiences of clients with the group counselling and what is their satisfaction with this counselling?
2. Have changes occurred in the clients who participated in the two different group-counselling programmes and if so, what are they and to what do the clients attribute the change or changes?
3. What is the relationship of the findings of these groups to the results obtained from other therapy evaluation studies?[8]

A prior measurement took place in the light of questionnaires after the first meeting. These questionnaires were also completed directly after the course ended[9] (the checking) and a year after the counselling ended (the follow-up). This last research was also accompanied by a verbal interview. I will give a brief summary of a few results.[10] The average report mark given to the course 'Living in the vortex' was an 8 (80%), while the companion group scored a 8.4 (84%) here. Measurement of quality of life showed no significant difference in prior measurement, checking or follow-up. But symptoms were significantly diminished directly after the end of the course and were still so a year later. A significant improvement in general functioning, in joie de vivre and in optimism was experienced. There were also questions as to the giving of meaning and self-realisation.[11] There was indeed a positive change in experiencing meaning for the

7 *Ruimte voor jezelf: Evaluatie groepsbegeleiding voor mensen met kanker door het Helen Dowling Instituut* (Space for yourself: Evaluation group supervision for people with cancer by the Helen Dowling Institute), Utrecht 2000.

8 *Ruimte voor jezelf*, 17.

9 At that moment a 'then-measurement' was taken, where the clients were asked to look back at their functioning before the intervention. Ten items from the HDI-A and HDI-O of the *Health and Disease Inventories* were used.

10 For an extensive discussion of various researches into the Kabat-Zinn method, see K.E. Bras, 'Hoe heilzaam is meditatie voor mensen met psychische en fysieke klachten' (How salutary is meditation for people with psychological and physical complaints), in: *Bulletin voor Charismatische Theologie* (2005) no 56, 18-31.

11 This involved four statements: 'I am very limited in my self-development'; 'I do know what I want and I can realise that'; 'I know myself what my place in life is'; and 'I have enough time for myself'.

participants of the vortex course, but this change was not significantly great. Mood in general did not turn out to be significantly improved, although there was a clear decrease in feelings of depression. In summary the report states:

> A year after the end of the vortex course the average scores for the different well-being scales are lower than before it, indicating an improvement of symptom level and general functioning. Tension has been greatly reduced and there is a more optimistic attitude to life. No significant changes found relating to quality of life, being focussed on the illness, expressing emotions and experiencing meaning.[12]

Measuring spiritual experiences

Two HDI co-workers and a co-worker from the University of Amsterdam wrote an article about measuring spiritual experiences.[13] Previous research, also among cancer patients, has shown that spirituality is an important element of someone's quality of life. 'People with a high "spirituality level" appear to be able to tolerate a high level of physical symptoms (pain and tiredness) and to retain the capacity of enjoying life thereby'.[14]

Spirituality can take the form of religiousness, but this is not necessary. And certainly in our secularised society we meet spirituality without involvement in a personal God. The heart of spirituality is experiencing meaningfulness and the feeling of connection. Experiencing a higher power is also seen by many, but not by everyone, as a core element.

After having presented this concept framework, there is discussion of a number of spirituality questionnaires used in psychological research in the US. Few turned out to be suitable, for example because no distinction was made between spirituality and religiousness. Further, the psychometric research was scant. It was hoped that the elements given in the model would offer a clearer point of departure for a new questionnaire to be formulated.

The Behouden Huys

The Behouden Huys in Haren, The Netherlands (www.behoudenhuys.nl) is an initiative of the professors Tjerk Hupkes and Rob Wesdorp. Both were cancer patients who had developed the CD-ROM 'You can live with cancer'. This has been distributed between 40,000 cancer patients for free in the meantime. The

---

12 *Ruimte voor jezelf*, 61.

13 B. Garssen, D. van Dierendonck & S. Tromp, 'Meten van spirituele ervaringen: Aspecten van en vragenlijsten over spiritualiteit' (Measuring spiritual experiences: Aspects and questionaires on spirituality), in: *Gedrag & Gezondheid* (Behaviour and Health) 29 (2001) no 4, 211-227.

14 *Ibid.*, 212.

Behouden Huys is a psycho-oncologic therapy centre: an institute that helps cancer patients to find their own way. It is situated in a wonderful new building on a country estate just outside the built up area of Haren. Large windows look out onto the woods, there is a lot of light, and the furnishings are tasteful and in light pastel colours. There are small interview rooms and large group rooms. There is an information counter by the entrance and further along there is an open space containing a large table with literature on it. There is a wide variety of items on the programme, ranging from one-off information evenings and personal counselling to courses on 'learning to live with cancer', 'inner healing', 'stress reduction' and a weekly open meditation morning.

I have had discussions with those who lead the meditation morning and the stress reduction course, and with a number of participants in the meditation morning. The names of the latter are replaced by fictitious names, to guarantee their privacy.

The meditation morning

The weekly meditation morning is lead by Prem Hannah Winkler. She has had experience with diverse forms of meditation since 1979, such as the dynamic mediation of Baghwan, Zen meditation, Vipasanna meditation. She has taken a ten-day training five times given by Goenka, a master from India, among other things. Meditation has been a daily practice for her for years, in which she primarily learned to be in stillness with herself, to go inside. She was brought up in the Hervormd Church, but is no longer connected to a church. Yet she is indeed religious in spite of this. 'What I profoundly experience in meditation, I can give no other name than "God"'. She got cancer a while ago. During that time she became involved with the Behouden Huys as a client. In the meantime, she is a member of the client advisory board and she has been supervising the meditation morning since May 2002.

In her opinion, the significance of meditation for people's wellbeing is that one learns to be quiet with oneself, learns to find strength within oneself and learns to make choices that one thinks are important. 'Death has touched us. Through meditation you learn to live, to seek another quality of life, yes, and you also learn to die. You do this by relaxing yourself, making contact with your body and being conscious of what is happening with you and in you. You learn to make contact with love. Love for yourself, love for the other'.

The meditation mornings that are given every week are not designed as a course, but can be visited one at a time. The number of people present varies from five to twelve. The relationship man/woman is about 3/7, ages between 40 and 60 years old. The participants suffer from cancer, or are partners of the patients. Most of them had an intake interview on their first contact with Behouden Huys. It was then discussed with them which counselling best suited them. They often take the course 'Learn to live with cancer' or another course, in addition to visiting the meditation.

The sessions last for 2 hours. Afterwards people meet each other in another space with a cup of coffee or tea. The meditation has different components. It begins with a relaxation exercise, often from the autogenic training. Afterwards a poem is read aloud and music is listened to in silence for ten minutes. There is a subsequent fifteen minutes of silent meditation, whereby people may sit as they wish, and they are taught how to use breath as an anchor point for thoughts that wander too much. Finally there is a moment of sharing with each other, without any obligation to say anything. Although this is not a therapy group and the discussion has not a dominant position, many people do find that it is a valued component of the meditation morning.

There is no targeted aftercare. But most participants experience the Behouden Huys as their 'home' and take part in other programmes or ask for personal counselling if they need it. There is empathy for out of the ordinary developments, a memorial service is held for those who die and there is a bereavement group for surviving next of kin.

No research has been done into the effects of meditation, but from the feedback people give, it would seem that they regard it as exceptionally positive.

The Behouden Huys is neutral regarding philosophy of life. 'But we treat people's spiritual and religious outlooks and experiences with much respect and openness. If they wish to contribute these it is always discussible. I myself sometimes experience so intense a happiness in meditation that only the word "God" covers it'.

The stress reduction course

Irène Bakker gives the stress reduction course. She has been involved in Zen meditation since 1986, became a Buddhist in 1989 and since 1995 has been a priest in the Zen tradition. She was trained full time in Zen for seven years in America, and before and after this had taken training courses in Europe and the US. She is dharma holder in the Lineage of Genpo Merzel Roshi. She began Kabat-Zinn's stress reduction method in Salt Lake City in 1998. Although this method is grounded in *Vipasanna* meditation, she sees great similarities with Zen. Although the schools are strictly separate in the East, people in the West seek to meet each other much more and also use methods from other traditions. One may choose a form of concentration meditation such as koan meditation in the Rinzai school of Zen or, as in *Vipasanna*, concentrate on that which comes to their attention, investigate it and then let it go. Or, as in the Soto school of Zen, one can let all thoughts come and go in an open alertness. It all comes down to an open form of consciousness in the end.

Irène gives workshops at home and abroad on dealing with dying, Zen meditation, and also a course called 'Fear, Zen and joie de vivre'. She has been leading the stress reduction course in the Behouden Huys since 2002. She views the significance of meditation for people's wellbeing as follows: 'Meditation can bring you to yourself. Who are you really? You are more than someone with cancer or with problems. Meditation helps you to very much live in the now. It is helpful in valuing life, and living to the full. Meditation is also a great help in illness. In times of crisis the necessity of walking a spiritual path comes to the fore very much. For your whole world is turned upside down. You are then open for something new. You can gain insight through meditation – inner wisdom and compassion. Compassion for yourself and for others. Illness can thus be a chance for a new perspective on life and death. Moreover it works very practically, as a good remedy against stress. This is not about stress disappearing. Stress goes with living. This is about learning to deal with it differently, so that you can manage the stress, and partly through this relaxation occurs'.

Ten people are participating in her group at the moment, four men and six women. They are aged between forty and sixty with one younger person. The symptoms with which they came to the course are the result of cancer, and have to do with the tension that accompanies the illness, also in the social sphere. People want to get to know their own limitations and so learn to live with them. They want to learn how to express themselves honestly.

There are also existential questions: what do I want to do with the time remaining to me? Questions on giving meaning and significance are of vital interest. 'As a Zen priest, I am of course open to them. I hope to be able to contribute to them finding a new manner of conscious life, but I am not doing missionary work. We do not always know what philosophy of life the clients have as background, but we are open and respectful to it and if it is broached, then it is certainly discussible in the group'.

She usually has a personal intake interview with every aspiring participant, although for all sorts of reasons that didn't happen with this group. She advises people with psychotic symptoms or symptoms of extreme depression against taking part.

The course takes place once a week for eight weeks, for two and a half-hours each time. She follows the Kabat-Zinn method plan. This means that one practises the body scan, yoga and seated meditation. One is given these exercises on a CD to take home too and is expected to practice each day for three-quarters of an hour. But she also adds some things to this method on occasion, such as a walking meditation in the wonderful woods surrounding the Behouden Huys. There is one more return day for the participants a month after the course. The aftercare then just occurs quite naturally, because the clients feel at home here and often participate in other programmes or get personal counselling.

No research has as yet been done into the effects of the course. The participants do fill in an evaluation form, where they usually indicate that they think about the course very positively. Talks are in progress with the academic hospitals in Groningen about beginning this kind of research. Further there is contact with both hospitals in Groningen and with hospitals in Assen and Hoogeveen.

Meditation for Irène is a way to deep consciousness, being part of a greater entity, call it 'transcendence'. 'Meditation can in this way bring you to a completely different view of life, a sense of connection with everything, with the universe, whatever you want to call it. I would wish it for everybody. But, as I said, I am not here to win souls. It is always discussible'.

Participants in the meditation morning: Margreet

Margreet is 57 years old. Three years ago she turned out to have a rare and serious form of cancer. An operation got rid of a growth in the abdomen, but new secondary tumours keep on occurring, in unexpected locations. She recently had to have a stoma fitted. She used to lead an extremely busy life as manager of a company. She was always ready to jump in and help others, but never considered her own needs. 'I have saved various marriages for my employees, but I've married and divorced twice myself'. Looking back she asks herself whether that lifestyle perhaps contributed to her becoming ill. Since her illness her life has changed radically. 'Then I was only partly living, because I never took the time to explore my deeper self. Now I feel much more one unity'. When she was in hospital she looked out upon some trees. One of the trees looked very mangled. It had been pruned very drastically in an ugly way. 'That is what I am now', she thought. That released an enormous rage in her. 'I am not going to be ground down. I want to live!' When she was discharged she bought a recreation house in the woods and lived in its tranquillity for a year. Trees began to mean much to her. 'If I touched them, a power emanated from them'. She realised that she had to do it herself. 'Of course your children and other people can help you, but you still have to do it yourself'.

Because she sought rest, and help for insomnia, she began to practice meditation, read spiritual books and came into contact with a man who helped her further on her spiritual path.

A year ago her son brought the Behouden Huys to her attention and she signed on for the basic course. She has been going to the meditation mornings for some time now. She primarily seeks rest in meditation. She is always busy doing a lot of things at the same time. This makes it difficult for her to concentrate. She wants to find a balance in herself and also learn to keep her body under control. She experiences the meditation as very positive, thinks it is wonderful to meditate with a group and exchange experience. She also needs the stimulus of the counsellor. She enjoys the music and the silent meditation the most. In the future she would like to confront her cancer more, by visualising it and physically combating it.

At present she feels reasonably well. She has good medication for the pain. 'You push back the frontiers more and more. I used to get much more panicky when I felt pain, but I have learned to look at my fears. Meditation helps with this, because you learn that fear says more about yourself. Why are you afraid? What can you yourself do about it? Can you learn to see the positive? What do you still have?'

The meditation strengthens this learning process in her. 'I now listen to my body much more, I no longer run away from fears. I'm no longer afraid of death. I do want to keep on living, but when the end comes, I am at peace with that too. I learn to value myself through meditation. Only a part of me used to live. Now I feel complete. I had no compassion for myself and knew no inner peace. Now I do. And that has also physical consequences. Because of it I am a medical miracle, actually. Three years ago the doctors thought I had only three months, and look, I'm still here'.

She has also grown spiritually, thanks to meditation. 'I was not brought up very religiously. As a child I went to Sunday school. But I have always been sensitive to it. It became more of an issue when I lived in the wood for that year. Trees give me strength. I am also very sensitive to smell. I am already longing to smell the scent of the earth when spring comes soon. Sometimes it is difficult. Recently after an operation I thought that I would die. I was completely ready for it. Then I did recover again and had to start again. You have to begin over again. And yet, I feel a certain sort of strength that helps me go on'.

Loes

Loes is a 54-year old woman. 'I was diagnosed with breast cancer in August 1998. A breast was amputated, lymph nodes were removed and then a bone marrow transplant, chemotherapy and radiation followed. After this I suffered extreme tiredness and had to give up my job as an executive secretary. I was taking lessons in Tai Chi before I came into contact with the Behouden Huys. But I had to deal with so much that I needed further counselling. After a period of individual psychotherapy I signed on for a course called "Learning to live with cancer" in the Behouden Huys. My GP had told me about this centre. I had already worked with the CD-ROM and so was already familiar with forms of meditation. I found sharing your experiences with others in a group of fellow sufferers an enormous enrichment. After the basic course I took the follow-on course, now take part in the meditation and have recently started taking the stress reduction training. I am also active in the client advisory board'.

What does she seek in meditation? To become more in touch with herself, to find rest in herself, to learn to be clearer about what she does or does not want, can or can not do in her social contacts. She has noticed that the weekly meditation is not enough for her. She looks for a point of rest every day and does a relaxation exercise. She experiences the meditation mornings as peaceful, familiar. 'You don't share your experiences as intensively as in the basic course, but that isn't the point either. I always enjoy it, whether it's the relaxation exercise now, or the poem or the music on another occasion, or the silent meditation that appeals to me'.

Partly through the meditation she has learnt to deal with the limitations the illness brings, such as the loss of her work. She experienced the effect of the meditation very practically during an examination she was recently subjected to. 'When I had been lying in the scan for three-quarters of an hour, I used the body scan exercise that I had learnt in the stress reduction training, and that helped me immensely at that moment. There are people who become panicky from lying in the scan. I have notice that I can deal with it better because of the meditation'. She thinks that her life has been very changed through her illness, but also through a changed attitude, mainly changed for the better! 'I used to be always busy, with my work, my family and then a course of studies as well. That stress charges you with all sorts of negative feelings. By illness forced me to start living differently. That was difficult, but through the meditation I have learned to deal with disappointments and to manage my stress better. I have found the strength to go on and to look at the positive. I have also learned to dose out my energy better, even if you sometimes go over your limits. You shouldn't look at what you can no longer do, but what you still can do. I have become more clear to myself too, I now see my limitations more sharply and I also sometimes dare to say no'.

Loes had been originally Reformed Church, but had not done much in connection with that any more. She married a man who was not a believer and partly because of this she had no contact with a church for years. However, when she was very ill indeed after the bone marrow transplant she felt as if she was being carried by a spiritual reality. She was deeply touched by this and this led to her now regularly visiting ecumenical services in Groningen and actively working on this. Preparing a religious address and the singing too, means a lot to her. The meditation has a positive effect on her spirituality. 'I am learning to love myself, I am allowed to be as I am, through this I learn to value others more, to see the divine in every person. That gives an enormous feeling of connection. And that again has a positive effect on how you feel, physical and spiritually'.

Jany

Jany is 58 years old. Six years ago she turned out to have breast cancer. She was treated then, effectively as she thought. But in 2002 she turned out to have new metastasis. She went though chemotherapy, which was very heavy, but ultimately seemed successful. Until the condition reared its head again a little while ago. She now feels that this is the beginning of the end. Her life has changed drastically as a result of the illness. She was an executive secretary, but is now on sickness benefit. Her husband left her three years ago which was an enormous blow to her. But she has started thinking about things because of all this. 'If you get something like this, then it's saying something to you. You have to discover what it is'. Jany busied herself with Simonton therapy, whereby you tackle your illness with meditative visualisations among other things, and with 'attitudinal healing' that uses supervised meditations. All this lead to increased consciousness, that you have to stick up for yourself and that mental power can mean much if you are ill.

'I wasn't brought up religiously, it was even anti-religious, actually. But due to the attitudinal healing I became more involved with the spiritual. I started thinking about death differently. There has to be something after death, but what?'

When the illness returned after the latest chemotherapy, she sought contact with the Behouden Huys. She has been taking the basic course since October 2002, and has attended the meditation mornings a number of times. What did she expect of this? 'I'll see what happens. I'm always like that, I never expect tangible things, I always wait and see. But I did hope to find inner peace and inner wisdom. Hope that I could get in touch with myself and with my inner leader'.

She experienced the mornings as very honest, and enjoyed the stillness, but has always had trouble preventing her thoughts from wandering. She also regularly meditates at home. Then she lies on the bed and imagines a place where she feels at home, usually in nature. Then she lets sunlight come into her and fill her completely. That helps her to let things go. What she likes about a group is the supervision. That stimulates you to get going with meditation. Wen she meditates at home by herself she sometimes misses that stimulus.

She actually does not know how she is doing at the moment. To what degree the illness will manifest in the near future is not certain.

In her experience the meditation helps her. 'It gives me tranquillity in my self. I used to have a lot of difficulty with my body. I was afraid of what was happening in my body. Now I can accept my body much more. Meditation helps me to accept that it is all right as it is. I was always escaping. I always ran away from my feelings and from my vulnerability. Because of the Simonton therapy and meditation, I now know and feel that I have to listen to myself really well, which among other things involves guarding my boundaries much better and not letting others stampede over me. And that has made me much more secure. Meditation helps me to put things in perspective. I can still get annoyed at other people's behaviour, but I really have learned to put it in perspective a bit more. I do think humour is very important in my situation. I used to be so afraid of death, but I don't have that anymore. I think that dying doesn't have to be that difficult. When my mother died she actually passed away very gently. Wouldn't dying be like that: that your spirit very slowly releases itself from the body? I hope so. And then? I don't know that precisely. It might be that you merge into the whole, or that you return in order to go on in the school of life. I don't know. But I do believe that there is something'.

'I do believe in a kind of God, although I wasn't brought up religiously. But what I do not believe in is sin and punishment. I absolutely do not believe in that. Meditation certainly has a spiritual significance for me, although I do occasionally deal with it in a forced way. I'm always frightened to fail at the crucial moment. That hampers me occasionally in meditation. Then I think that I'm not able to get to that peace that I seek. But I once had a special experience. We had to take various "steps" during a meditation in order to turn inward into ourselves, and I thought again: Can I do it? And suddenly it came over me: I was one with all things, I felt myself connected to everything around me. I can't call up an experience like that again, I think that's a pity sometimes, but I haven't forgotten it. Yes, meditation really means something to me. It gives me a sense of peace. And that is what I seek'.

Participants in the stress reduction training: Anke and Johan

When I arrive, I am let into a house undergoing conversion. New building work has been done too: a new kitchen and a wonderfully light sun room. 'This is being built for the future', I think, 'a house for light'.

Anke is 56 years old and her husband Johan is 57, sympathetic to and involved in religion. In the course of their lives they had already developed a great deal, whereby they were each occupied in their own way with newer theological insights and forms of spirituality. He is more a do-er, she more a thinker. She was used to regularly retreat to her room for a quiet moment, by a candle and an icon, was interested in mysticism and also followed a few meditation courses in monasteries. They both also went to meetings of the charismatic movement, and in the ecumenical monastery of Taizé.

In August 2000 Anke turned out to have cancer. Her doctor initially made light of the situation, but her intuition told her that this was not all right. She was operated on and she turned out to have an aggressive form of gynaecological cancer with several metastasis. After the operation, a long period of chemotherapy followed, which made her completely bald. She felt herself become more and more sick in this six months of chemotherapy. She also had, understandably, to come to terms with a heavy mental blow. She functioned increasingly badly, could not walk for more than ten minutes and needed domestic help. Johan had just begun new work that demanded a lot of his attention, yet now he had a lot of additional domestic matters and the shared worries also took their toll. Anke sometimes felt so sick that she thought: 'I don't want to go on any more!' But she resisted this apathy by calling in the words of Jesus that he said to a man who had been sick for many years: 'Do you wish to become healthy?' And she thought in addition to this: 'And will you do anything for this yourself?' That helped her to go on fighting for her future at any rate. She had had some strange experiences too, just before she discovered that she was sick. On holiday in the tent she had an image in her mind of someone who was completely bald and wrapped up. Another time, one night, she saw that the tent was surrounded in light, while her husband saw nothing. The sense that the light would lead her through this darkness, strengthened her in difficult moments. The illness had far reaching effects socially too. She could share everything very openly with the children. They were a very close warm family.

On the other hand there were also people, especially in her work circle, from whom she had expected support but who bitterly disappointed them. Happily there was also a friendly preacher who regularly visited them; he gave Anke extreme unction several times, whereby she once say a light surrounding her at that moment. Exceptional experiences that comforted and encouraged them. Yet Anke had a sense that she had to seek help to come to terms with the heavy physical and mental blow. 'Everything in my life was turned upside down', she said.

She saw a Behouden Huys folder and sent away for the CD-ROM 'You can live with cancer'. After a while she sought contact and took the basic course and the follow-up course. Bernie who counselled her, said to her later: 'When you came here fear was radiating from you'. It was mainly the fear of death, but also all sorts of other fears. 'My deepest fear was that I would end up alone, that people would drop me. Luckily Johan never did that. As a woman, you also ask yourself if you are still attractive to him with your bald head. But he was always sweet and mild. But I did make it very difficult for myself. When I was bald I couldn't look in the mirror for a year actually. It was then wonderful to experience that you can just be yourself in the Behouden Huys, that you can say anything, that there is no judgement expressed. Once more I was able to experience how much love and warm involvement you can receive from a group of people that you did not know before. You were allowed to just be with everything you have, and you need that very much in such a situation. You need closeness and sympathy, and I got that there'.

After the basic course and the follow-up course she signed up for the stress reduction course, together with her husband. Johan had once been to an information evening for partners and now there was a chance to do a course as partner he grasped that with both hands. Not only because he could empathise with

Anke in this way, but he himself needed support. They were difficult years for both of them, also because many deaths and illnesses occurred in their broader family. 'I was looking for handles in order to live in a more disciplined meditative manner', he said, ' for only in this way would I be able to keep going. I had read many books about it but now I wanted to experience it from the inside'. 'And I', said Anke, 'I was looking for myself. I wanted to find myself again, as happy and balanced as I was before my illness. Although I have gradually discovered that that is unrealistic. I have been changed forever through this whole process. But in any case I wanted to work on my mental pain, my instability, my stress'.

The stress reduction course consisted of eight sessions and a reprise day. Fixed elements were the body scan, yoga and seated meditation. They got three CDs to take home and practice and did so regularly. They both experienced this course as very healing. Johan: 'I have learned to live in the here and now, to let go of the future and the past more, to really focus your attention on the situation you are in at this moment. That way you also really learn to give one hundred percent attention to the person you are dealing with now. Sometimes the exercises at home were so relaxing that I fell asleep. It was new to me that mind and body are so connected to each other'. Anke was not able to participate so much in the yoga exercises because of a painful arm, but she then again learned with the help of the body scan to go to the painful place with her attention, and that often gave some relief. 'I mainly learned what it is to live in an attentive way, and without making judgements. Doing this gives you compassion for yourself, and you find a place in yourself where peace and faith live. You learn to let things go, principally to let go of the grip on yourself'.

How are her symptoms at the moment? Anke: 'I am now more resistant to stress. In the beginning if you have been overcome by illness, you are very vulnerable. I absolutely couldn't stand it if someone talked to me loudly. You shut yourself off because you are hurt. I gradually got more confidence which has made me more resistant to stress, although I will have to develop further here. I've also learned not to look too far into the future, but to live more in the here and now. And I am functioning much better, I can even walk for three-quarters of an hour, I get tired less quickly'. She is very clearly convinced that the meditation has helped her. She feels much stronger physically, even if that is strength in weakness. She can manage the pain in her arm better using the attention training and has also learned to recognise and acknowledge her boundaries through it. She has also become stronger psychologically. 'I am much more aware of myself, with more respect for myself and fellow human beings, I now realised the value of dealing carefully with others. If I get into a difficult situation, I have now learned to withdraw into a quiet place in myself. I place a reassuring image in front of my eyes, for instance a water lily on the water, that openness, that surrender, that release, and then that helps me. I have also learned not to let myself be determined by what others think and find, but to have myself as starting point, travel by my own compass'. Johan has also been helped by the course. 'Of course I didn't have the kind of physical symptoms that Anke had. It mainly had a psychological and social effect on me. Lovingly paying attention to people, the sense that everyone has a piece of individuality, that you can be completely there for someone else for a moment, I learnt that from Irène's example above all. I also learned from it how to find a rest point in yourself, how to release, to live in a less forced way, as well as compassion for yourself and others. Perhaps these things were in me already, but they were reinforced by the course'.

Changes happened on the spiritual level too. In the beginning that was primarily negative for Anke, partly because of disappointing experiences in her church circle, that left a kind of vacuum afterwards. 'For two years, I no longer retreated to my little room to meditate. I consciously distanced myself from the "pious life". It returned slowly, in particular because of the loving approach in the Behouden Huys. I have now come to see myself far more as a part of that divine whole, I have received eyes to see the light that falls into my life. I'm allowed to stand in the light again'. The unusual experiences she had just before the illness came to light and at the extreme unction reinforced this sense in her: 'I now experience God much more as full of love, more as involvement, a strength that helps me go on and leads, what ever may further happen. But I need to experience God in people around me. I missed that for a while, but it is beginning to come back again'.

Johan also speaks of the significance this whole process has had for his spiritual life. 'For me, God has increased in strength into a source, a basis for faith, whatever happens. God is less in words, more in stillness and perception. He is a source of light. Where love is, there is God. To experience this in the Behouden Huys with people of all sorts of different backgrounds has broadened my sense of God. The accent has also moved in my work from organisation to being more involved with people in a conscious, concerned way. And I believe that we both are able to have also compassion for those who have disappointed us'.

I then get a cup of soup and a roll. Right at the end Anke says to me: 'Do you know what I also learned? To accept death. And that's what gives me vitality. For if you are too busy with the fear of death, it costs you so much energy that you don't live life enough. I live far more consciously now, and also more gratefully. I can enjoy the small things. I can live in the light. That's why I wanted this sun room, because of the light'.

Conversations around the Taborhuis (Tabor House)

I visited the Taborhuis on Friday 14th February 2003. It is situated in Groesbeek, near Nijmegen.

The building used to be a doctor's house. It contains a number of smaller and large rooms, where there is a secretarial office and where it is possible to carry out personal interviews and meet with small groups. The programmes with larger groups are held in the hall, elsewhere in the grounds.

In 1990 the Taborhuis was founded as a centre for psychosocial counselling for people with cancer. In the meantime it has also opened itself to people with other life threatening illnesses such as MS and Aids. In the first place, counselling is personal in nature: patients, with or without their partners, talk to one of the counsellors – psychologists, psychotherapists, theologians, psycho-energetic therapists, physiotherapist, workers in social areas. This helps them to increase the quality of their lives, to deal with changes in their future prospects, to find balance again and to improve their social relationships. In addition, there is also the possibility of taking group meeting, including the meditation group I witnessed.

Psycho-energetic therapy
Psycho-energetic therapy, as developed by William Yang and Tom Staps, is the foundation of the work of the Taborhuis.[15] This therapy assumes the following model.[16]

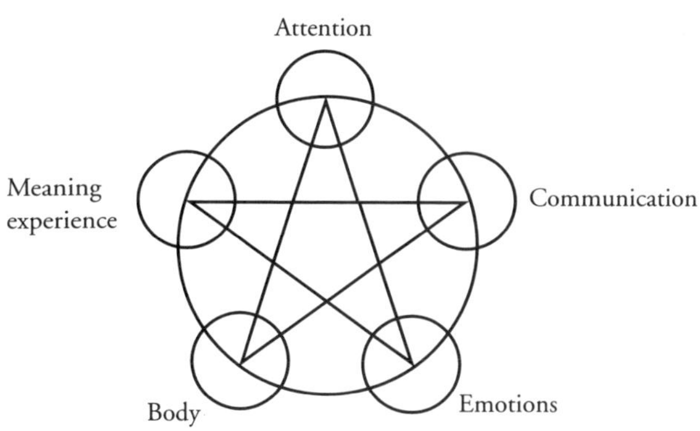

[15] And described in the book T. Staps & W. Yang, *Psycho-energetische therapie: Psychosociale begeleiding van kankerpatienten* (Psycho-energetic therapy: Psychosocial supervision of cancer patients), Nijkerk 1991.

[16] The model comes from Staps & Yang, *Psycho-energetische therapie*, 20.

Man is seen here as an open system, composed of subsystems of different levels and in connection with greater systems within which he must attempt to hold his ground in a continuous flow of inner and outer changes. Cancer is a serious disturbance of the system, which begins on the level of the body, but which also touches other aspects of human existence, as presented in this model. Conversely the other subsystems, such as attention, emotions etc., may also exert their influence upon the body. Psycho-energetic therapy is concerned with strengthening the flexibility, the mobility of the whole system by optimising communication between the different subsystems. The subsystem that the therapy takes as starting point depends on the patient. I will give a short impression of how one works on the level of the different subsystems.

Attention

Directing attention is practised, with the aim of freeing this, so that people gain a better control of their attention, and do not become continually obsessed with attention to the painful or sick place in the body, but also do not run away from it. People learn to release. 'Releasing requires a greater strength of mind than clinging on or doggedly resisting it. Releasing assumes another sort of strength, namely that of surrendering and the courage to walk an unknown path'.[17]

Communication

People communicate verbally, 'para-verbally' (emotions that resonate in for example the sound of the voice), and non-verbally. 'Open interaction and congruency between attention, verbal message, emotional and physical reaction; great openness to discussion of the personal situation, but likewise the capacity to reject this, if they feel this will disturb their balance; an ability to close themselves to information that will make dealing with their situation more difficult; readiness to explain lack of clarity', all this is encouraged in the therapy.[18]

Emotion

A threatening illness like cancer arouses strong emotions for the patient and his immediate circle. Learning to manage and deal with these emotions is an important facet of this counselling. This involves learning to recognise the emotion, to then express and examine it. Building a relationship of trust between patient and counsellor is important here. If useful and necessary, relaxation exercises and visualisations are deployed in the therapy in order to learn to acknowledge, to experience emotions and also to release them again.

---

[17] Ibid., 29.

[18] Ibid., 39.

Body

The body is an open subsystem of a human being. The other subsystems may have influence on physiological processes and on the body's experience. The therapy works on the experience of pain by finding in the body another anchor spot for itself than the painful place. Here this primarily involves forms of relaxation and release by means of breathing via the pelvis. Thus one does not only learn to direct attention to the body as a whole. But also to experience the body as included in a greater entirety.

Giving and experiencing of meaning

'If the patient succeeds in arriving at an effective provision and experience of meaning, he maintains the feeling of be able to cope with the situation and to have a directional influence upon it, even if he no longer has a grip on much of what occurs. He possess the will to make his situation meaningful, to deal with it as well as possible. He keeps his interests and makes plans as long as possible, even if the remaining time is very brief'.[19] Different ways of correcting the ineffective giving of meaning and promoting the effective giving of meaning are attempted in the therapy. One of the approaches is using meditation emphasising opening to a greater whole by means of the breath. 'The human being is no longer anxiously contained and isolated, but lets things pass through, transparent as it were'.[20]

Description of a group meeting

I enter the hall a little late, where the group under the leadership of William Yang began at 10 o'clock and are now sitting drinking tea. The room is rather ugly, old room with linoleum on the floor and a small stage. There are windows that do let light through but do not let us be seen. There are about twenty participants. They discuss how the exercises, which they took home on cassette tape, went during the past week. A little more information is given, about a Teleac (Television Academy) course for example and a few books. Afterwards we gather in a circle all made of mattresses lying on the ground with cushions on them. The participants have all brought a blanket or sleeping bag with them. There are exercises done while standing for the first half an hour. Mr Yang leads us through the exercises with a slight touch of humour and at an easy pace. We learn to concentrate on our feet in order to let go of the worries and thoughts in our head. A lot of flexibility and stretch exercises follow. Then we lie down on the mattress. Again, exercises which stretch the muscles and release them. Afterwards we

[19] Ibid., 87.

[20] Ibid., 91.

are asked to put our hands under our pelvis, with the palms of the hand downwards and the thumbs and fingers in a triangle around our sacrum. Then we focus our attention on this spot and breath in and out via this location in our pelvis. 'Breath in, not forcedly, just make space, then the breath flows in. Through this place energy flows inside you, energy from the cosmos. And let the energy flow through your body by every exhalation and give it back again. It is as if your sacrum has become completely porous, like that rock in the desert that Moses struck and then water came out of it. Inhale and then say softly to yourself "aah", like the sound of wonderment. And exhale and say to yourself softly "ooh" like a sound of surrender. Aah, ooh, like alpha and omega, ahh, ohh aaooem in Sanskrit'. Finally we go to sit in a circle, give each other a hand, breathe in and out softly, and pass the energy on to each other. Time is up, it is one o'clock again. I feel very deeply relaxed and have the impression that others are too. People stay and talk for a little while having tea. I go to the Taborhuis with William Yang for a conversation with him.

Conversation with William Yang

William Yang studied theology and sociology at the Catholic University of Nijmegen and in addition investigated psychotherapy during six summer vacations in the United States. During the study he led a centre for drama education. Afterwards he took a three-year ward orderly training course. After this course he lived for a year in China. He had become involved in meditation and yoga in the meantime. He was educated and trained by Robert van Hekeren, who was involved with meditation and social engagement, by Ilse Miedendorf, who taught him breath therapy in connection with Jungian psychotherapy, and above all by Hetty Draaier, through whom he made his own synthesis of Buddhism and Christianity. He has already often been in North India for periods of a few weeks, where he has contacts with Tibetan teachers, among them the Dalai Lama. In 1989 he started giving relaxation therapy to cancer patients, at the request of a specialist in the Canisius-Wilhelmina hospital in Nijmegen. He longed for his own place for this work, and this led to the foundation of the Taborhuis. It was originally accommodated in a wooden house in the Dekkerswald grounds, later it moved into the present premises. The organisation has grown with the years. There is now a director, Hetty Hendrikse, as well as nine therapists. When he was looking for a name for the centre, the name 'Tabor' arose, as a place of light. He later studied the significance of the Tabor in more depth. The transfiguration of Christ through the light of heaven has become for him the symbol of the transformation a person can undergo. Although Yang is a theologian and has given a name from the Christian tradition to this house, the centre is not based on Christian principles. No religious ideas or feelings are imposed during the group sessions, for the participants each have their own philosophy of life. Yet it is so that religious aspects are carefully, almost implicitly on offer, as struck me during the session. Hence, the suggestion is aroused that one communicates with a 'greater, healing entirety' through the breath. 'Yes', says Yang, 'I do suggest it, but very carefully so that everyone can interpret it according to his or her own views'.

He himself approaches meditation from feeling and enjoying the body. First of all attention goes to tension, in order to release it, then downwards, to release the worrying in the head, to the pelvis. The pelvis, and especially the triangle around the sacrum, is vitally important to finding a mid-point in your body. You find balance in yourself through this mid-point, but you also communicate with the world around you. Yang calls this 'the tabor eye'.[21] For him meditation is not only sitting still and breathing gently, but it is also movement, making sounds, sometimes even screaming and crying. He also gets people, often lying down, to become conscious of a 'refined physicality'. 'You are not only a material body, your body is also a living, energetic space, a breath space in which experiences become free'. Further he thinks it is also important to make a link between Buddhist attention for yourself and for repentance, and the Christian attention to your solidarity. Hence meditation is as much about insight as it is about love. 'In this way you feel yourself bedded down in that which is greater than yourself, greater than your sick body too. Through your own limited ego, you then come into something quite different. What is that? I do not want to interpret that too much for people, otherwise I would repel many'.[22]

The participants in the meditation group, a maximum of 20, are 15 percent men, eighty five percent women, with an average age of just over fifty. The group comes together weekly for two and a half hours, in blocks of three occasions. Then there is a week rest and it is possible to decide whether or not to participate in the following block. Some people have already been doing this for eighteen months to a year, others stop earlier for various reasons.

Research is being done into the effects of the entire supervision. A questionnaire with a quality of life scale and the scales of Antonovsky is completed. This research is repeated after three and after nine months. In general there is much

---

21 He wrote a leaflet in the 'Taborreeks' (Tabor series) with the title *Tabor: Visoen van het verheerlijkte lichaam* (Tabor: Vision of the exalted body). this leaflet is report of a journey he made in 1998 from the Tabor mountain to Bodhgaya, the place where Buddha attained enlightenment, via the Borobodur With the aid of a number of mandalas he presented a vision of the transformation of the human being, whereby the latter receives a part of the heavenly light by opening the cosmic eye, the triangle in the pelvis. He also recognises in the Hesychasm of Athos this attention to the entrance of the tabor light by concentrating in the middle of your body. Inner enlightenment and physical becoming whole thus fuse in a 'tantric Christianity'.

22 For more information on his manner of meditation see William Yang, *Yoga van moed en mededogen* (Yoga of courage and compassion), Groesbeek 1999.

satisfaction with the supervision and, and the component meditation scores an 8.5 (85%) on average.

Conversations with participants in the meditation sessions

My decision to travel to Nijmegen with the train was punished once again. One train was cancelled so that I arrived later than expected. I rang Marianne on my cell phone to say I was delayed. She offered to come and pick me up from the station, which I gladly accepted.

On the way to her house she told me that she had led the playgroup in the Taborhuis that morning. She was a drama teacher at a cabaret academy and has always worked a lot with all sorts of groups. Now she has disablement pension she thinks using her skills as a volunteer in a group of patients is wonderful. People get the opportunity to relate their experiences. Afterwards those experiences are given a theatrical form, where they are generalised into universally human experiences. This helps the members of the group to come to terms with their own experiences.

When we are sitting cosily around the table at her home and she has poured a cup of tea, she talks. She is 54 years old and lost her work in 1995 when she got a psychosis. She had already often been troubled by migraine and then the psychosis came along on top of this. She had to be hospitalised for a while. The diagnosis was made: manic depressive. It is an ailment that her mother, sister and brother have also experienced. 'My therapist advised me to do relaxation exercises. I then got a tape with exercises by William Yang and tried to do these exercises at home. At first I did them with great anxiety, that I would go and "fly" as we call it. We mean by this that you lose your contact with reality. But luckily that did not happen. And that's how it began with meditation'.

Marianne was brought up a strict Catholic. Her father had been a White Father. Her mother was Protestant, but became Catholic and as is frequently the case with 'converts', she was rather fanatic about this. 'I was brought up with all sorts of stories of the saints, in which there was incredible suffering for the greater honour and glory of God, and I was scared to death that God would also call me to become such a saint and have to suffer so much for my faith. Moreover the psychological disease worked itself out in my mother as a sort of religious delusion, and in the case of my brother it even took almost demonic traits. That frightened me off so much that I gave up my membership of the Church when I was eighteen. I had never heard that God a God of Love is'.

Shortly after Marianne had got to know about Yang's meditation method via her tape in 1995, she decided to take yoga lessons from him at the Han Fortmann centre. He asked her to assist him in the meditation course at the Taborhuis and now she takes part in the sessions and does odd jobs connected with them. She feels at home in the group, even although she herself does not have cancer. 'I can really identify with cancer patients because I also know what it is to have to let go all that you cling to. And also that you have to come to terms with an insecure future and with the idea that you have to organise your life differently'.

What did she expect from meditation when she began it? 'That the fretting in my head would stop. I was always preoccupied with my own problems. You look for a way out, but you don't find one. I hoped that I could empty my head by meditating. I suddenly felt so worthless because of my ailment and hoped that by meditating I could find sense of worth again. Perhaps I would become a good person because of it! I felt that I had completely lost control and had no self-confidence any more, and I hoped to regain that through meditation. I saw meditation as something that goes further than relaxation alone. And even although I was scared of the consequences of it in the beginning, luckily I went through with it and that has given me much. I have made it a practice to meditate daily, but the meditation group means a lot to me as well. The loving, compassionate, consenting atmosphere, that everything can just be! Experiencing this has strengthened the faith in me that I am supported, I have found a home in myself in the group. I have learned that I can release everything, for there is just ground under your existence. As William once said: "You still have your breath, and your sitting bones and the certainty that your breath will stop at some point". I enjoy the humour with which he leads the course and the approval in his attitude. I think it is important that you learn to let your attention drop from your head downwards, to your pelvis, and to your feet. It makes my head more spacious and lighter. I do think it is a pity that there is no lengthy silence, for that offers you the space to meditate yourself. That does happen on the monthly Monday mornings led by William Yang in the student chapel. They go deeper than the meditation in the Taborhuis, particularly because of the silence'.

The meditation has had clear effects on Marianne. She is far less troubled by migraine. Neither has she had any new psychosis since the episode in 1995 although she cannot ascribe this exclusively to meditation. Meditation has made her more able to fight. That was apparent when she recently heard that her son is suffering from schizophrenia. This is naturally very difficult for the whole family, but by meditating she was able to prevent herself from going into a depression about it and she can give her son a little bit of light too. She is now also going to work for the Pandora Foundation.

She also interacts with people differently because of meditation. 'I am less judgmental. If I see someone doing something that I don't like, I know that this often comes from defensiveness and fear and not from the fact that he is bad. I have become more compassionate, less strict. I go with the flow of events more. And crazily enough, I began to see nature. I never did that. I was a real city person, enjoyed pubs more than the woods. But now I started seeing nature! I saw the branches, and the buds and the removal of the buds and I saw through that as well. I started experiencing nature as a metaphor for our human existence. You could say that I entered into dialogue with Nature. I see the eternal value of it too. If I see a tree, I think: it has stood there for so long. I feel my own life absorbed into the flow of life and after my death I will be literally absorbed into that flow'.

Meditation has also had an effect on her experience of religion. 'Not that I believe again in a personal God. But if I see myself, others, Nature, then I cannot believe that that is just co-incidence. There has to be something behind it. And that is not only true of positive things, but also from the negative, the painful. There is a creative force at work, so that the creative process is always ongoing. And I too have a task in this. As a drama teacher I feel it in this way: I am the player and God is the director. I have to play my role. And I have to do that from inside out, by maintaining contact with what lives deeply inside me. I used to play for success, now for this self-realisation. And I believe that I contribute something to the greater whole like this, although I cannot point to it in any tangible way. I feel a faith that I serve some purpose. I have always had the feeling that I wanted to get to the invisible and I experience that in meditation'.

Conversation with Elise

While tea was being made, I looked around me in the cosy little conservatory where I had been planted. Many books, two little statues of the Buddha, a set of spiritual insight cards. She put a few drawings into my hands that her father had made and that are printed on the mourning circular and the liturgy of his funeral now. Drawings of the little church where the requiem mass was also held. He had recently passed away, a creative man, who did not only draw but also composed. 'And a kind man too', she said. 'We used to go to that church until my brothers said that they didn't want to any more. I took confirmation classes for a year, but afterwards I never went again either. But I didn't have an aversion to it. My father was very moderate in his faith, didn't impose anything on us. My mother was a real follower of Dorothee Sölle, a feminist'. Suddenly her eyes are full of tears. 'My mother got dementia. She could no longer stay living in their house. Before the funeral I read a poem to her. I had to weep. Then my mother said: "But that is beautiful poem. You shouldn't cry because of it". Look, she can do that, still suddenly say something like that'. She gave me the poem. I'm allowed to put it into my report.

Dieu essuiera toutes tes larmes
(God will dry all your tears)

A piece of music by Messiaen.
One of his last compositions
The light falls through the notes.
What a comfort.

Whoever God is.

Is he Space?
Is he the radiant light from within?
Is he the Comfort?
Is he Love between people?

Or is she a forget-me-not in the sun?
A Buddha that rises from middle?
A streak of coloured light in the air?
An tender, attentive glance?

Or perhaps a pebble in my shoe?
A quarrel with the children?
An illness in my body?
A sudden death?

No one will ever know.

Belief, trust, experience
That something or someone is around you and in you:
The Light, the Sun, the Space, the Cosmos, God's love
That carries you or guides you to your final destination.

Elise is a woman of fifty, social worker, still working as a supervisor. In January 200, she had a lump in her breast. It was initially considered not malignant by the GP and various specialists, but she remained uneasy. 'My intuition told me that things were not all right. Then I was finally operated on and I turned out to really have cancer after all. It was a mild form, however. After a lumpectomy and 32 radiation treatments I had completed treatment. Directly after the diagnosis of cancer I decided to go into therapy. Because I wanted to prevent myself becoming depressed. I had already been doing yoga for seven years, and afterwards began Tai Chi, but I was troubled by articular degeneration, so that this became more difficult. I was looking for another form and someone referred me to the Taborhuis counselling. I had conversations with William Yang. He made me personal tapes with meditation exercises that I could do at home. I do this twice a day now, and in addition I have been a member of the meditation group since April 2001'. Her articular degeneration symptoms were of such a nature that closer investigation was required. It became apparent that she suffered from hemochromatosis, an inherited illness where iron is retained by the body. She now has to regularly undergo bloodletting, which puts great demands on her energy. So she often suffers from serious fatigue. Moreover the articular degeneration resulting from this illness, has progressed to her hips, knees and ankles. She walks with difficulty, has a lot of pain and is waiting for two successive operations for new hips. 'It was a real blow to me, after the cancer to have this illness as well. In addition the dementia process in both parents and the death of my father demanded a lot of me'.

The meditation is a real support to her. The relaxation exercises allow the tension to come out. She needs her daily meditation, but in addition likes to meditate in the group as well. The group and William Yang's contribution inspire her. Aside from daily practice at home and the weekly meditation group in the Taborhuis. She also participates in the monthly meditation mornings that Willam Yang organises in the student chapel in Nijmegen. 'There is far more stillness there. There is no talking, there is more room to come to one's own meditation in stillness. And I need that. I need time to be able to release things and become empty'.

'I get a lot of images when meditating. I see things. In the beginning these were symbols of death, such as pyramids and megaliths. But recently I had this image: I stood before a sea. At the edge Jesus stood. The sea opened up. When I thought about this later, I understood what this wanted to say: that I'm allowed to go from the land of slavery to the promised land. And that is, that I can get more in contact with myself. I cannot call up these images by myself. If I keep on staying in my head, I don't get them. But if I can let everything go, then they are given to me'.

What effect did meditation have on her functioning? She hadn't noticed that it directly helped much physically. On the contrary, she has deteriorated further during the last year. But meditation does help her to relax and hence she has been able to deal with pain better. She has mainly noticed the effect in the mental sphere. She has not become depressed, and even if she is often tired and also sad, she can deal with it. 'You get strength from somewhere. I gain courage from the sense that you can drill for this strength yourself. Of course your body is your body, but your mind is so much more important. That I'm only able to work part-time for a few hours has not made me insecure or vulnerable as a person. I have also learned to live with death, and I can only do that in contact with a special power, a power that you can call on through meditation.' That brought us to spirituality. Elise broke with the church at the age of 24. 'For years I did not concern myself with faith. I'm also a born doubter. I don't take on something quickly and am not easily deeply convinced of something. But due to my illness, and to the meditation, it has come to the fore much more now. A remark of William's meant a lot to me. When I told him that I was finding it very difficult that my parents had dementia, that I was on the road to losing them, he said: "You are a child of *God* too". Do I now have faith? As an inveterate doubter I wouldn't easily say that. I am on the road, somewhere between Buddhism and

Christianity. I have only dared to let the word "God" pass my lips in the last two or three months. It is now becoming very important to me that God is love. You can read it in the poem that I wrote for my father's funeral and that I read aloud in the Tabor group'.

'I am not afraid to die. But I really want to check things, to plan. I am now learning to let that go. Things occur as they occur. You have to release and look at what there is. That's what I learn from meditating. That's why Buddhism appeals to me, that you also refer to the here and now. In society, it's keep on running in order to get more. I have let go of that obsession with the material. I would rather be'.

I am reminded of the closing words of her poem: *God's love/ That carries or guides you to your final destination.*

Conversation with Hanneke

Hanneke has her own practice as hypnotherapist and gestalt therapist and also does work as a social-psychiatric nurse. We conducted our conversation in her consulting room, where a few wonderful works of art hang on the wall, made by a close acquaintance who is very preoccupied with the spiritual and expresses that in her work. Hanneke is 53. She was operated on for breast cancer in November 2001. It was initially to be a lumpectomy, and then it turned out that the whole breast had to be amputated. There were also a few metastases in the lymph nodes so that she had to undergo radiation. 'I actually had a new blow to come to terms with each time, and I found that very difficult. I also thought it was very unfair. For I had stopped my work as a social psychiatric nurse and was busy looking for other work. I felt that I was on the right road and now suddenly this! I felt confused, and guilty too, I had the feeling that I hadn't lived well'. Hanneke was brought up in the Dutch Reformed Church, but hasn't been involved in the church for years. Although she did respect people who had a faith. She also didn't want any swearing in her family. 'I was angry with religion for a while. When I was doing my Nursing B training, I came across a lot of people who had become mentally ill through their faith. I thought then that many people were unnecessarily burdened with guilt feelings because of faith. But the anger was a just a passing phase. I wasn't brought up in a strict religious atmosphere. My father always held the way open for our children'.

The hypnotherapy training and the one for gestalt therapy and psychosynthesis brought her more in contact with that which is more profound, but yet still she closed herself off from this. When it was apparent that she had cancer, the longing emerged for... 'I was actually seeking happiness. I was actually not really happy. I would never send a New Year's card with "Happy New Year", for I always thought "what is happiness actually"? I thought that I sought a way to *grant* myself happiness. Moreover I was very tired after the radiation and sought a method of dealing with it. I also wanted to come into balance, become more stable'. All reasons why she chose meditation. She had heard about the Taborhuis indirectly and went to take personal counselling and the meditation group there shortly after her operation at the end of 2001. She hoped to come home to herself through the meditation, to be more herself and she longed to be more who she is. She also wanted to give the cancer and the meditation more of a place in her life. And these expectations were not disappointed. 'I experience being allowed to rest, I'm allowed to be, and talking is allowed, but you don't have to. I learn how to surrender to what is good for myself. Recently I have been trying to get up the discipline to meditate at home and I notice that it is becoming more familiar, more something that belongs to me. I can also apply what I learn there in daily life. For example, if a client comes to my practice, then I first do a short breathing exercises. I feel more peaceful then, and well prepared. I get a lot of benefit out of it'.

She enjoys the 'divine' in the meditation most of all, in the way she experiences this in the Taborhuis. 'If you can say ooo to the rhythm of your breath, then I feel in it the words clean, and god, and cosmos, and if that "ooo" then becomes "aum", then I feel how that connects everything to everything. I once also had a deep experience during the meditation, I was there, I wasn't floating, I was very awake, I felt completely at one with myself, and one with everyone and everything, with something very magnificent. Suddenly I didn't feel my body any more. I also felt an intense peace. I felt that this was my home. I would like to have an experience like that once again, but you can't call it up. And, to a less intense degree, I do often feel the same in essence. That gives me faith in life and in going on. Only I just don't know if I want to call the source that you then experience God or the Divine. God as a person, I think that's too limited. Moreover it calls up memories in me of all sorts of things that weren't allowed. In "the Divine" I feel far more the source of strength that dwells deep within me. Someone recently called that "spirit strength", and perhaps that is a good expression for it. I now go to church occasionally and then I can sing the hymns again. I used to not be able to get the words out of my mouth, but now I see what is behind them more. You know, we sometimes sing in the meditation group, and that is sometimes very emotional. Yes, I have now returned to God, but now I believe in a really good way, a very accepting way, without the guilt I used to have'.

Hanneke expressed these things in a thoughtful way, as if she still had to get used to them herself. Her physical symptoms have improved. She does have trouble with her arm, but it doesn't rule her life any more. She has settled down and can deal with her energy much better. She has learned to accept her amputation. Initially she felt her breast prosthesis as something false, now the breast prosthesis is just part of her. She feels whole, in spite of her breast prosthesis.

Meditation teaches you to love yourself, your own body too, you learn to value yourself, she said. 'I knew all this already, naturally through my work and training too, but I am now really feeling it through the meditation. I feel myself becoming more and more complete'.

Attendance at the Attention Training

My research into the literature as well as my visit to the three centres mentioned showed that the attention training/stress reduction training as developed by Kabat-Zinn, is frequently applied and appears to be effective. So I took a similar training myself. This was given by Johan Tinge, psychotherapist,[23] and consisted of eight afternoon sessions of two and half hours and an additional full day. Moreover we aimed at doing three quarters of an hour of exercises every day during which we were guided by cassette tapes. These exercises consisted of the body scan (go through the whole body in minute detail with complete attention), yoga in a prone and a sitting position, and sitting meditation. In addition to these formal exercises, we were also given more informal instructions on how to live attentively and instructions aimed at increasing our insight into dealing with stress. The formal and informal exercises were outlined in an 'attention training course workbook' that we had received. I will now give an overview of the sessions and a short summary of my own experiences.

First week

There were eight participants, four women and four men. Course leader Johan Tinge first gave some practical information. Then there was a round of introductions. Roughly half of those taking part suffer from psychological symptoms, like depression. Two have physical symptoms and two, including myself, were mainly taking part for professional reasons.

We did a few attention exercises, including the body scan (paying attention to your feeling in various body parts lying down on a mat for half an hour). We did the body scan at home every day with the aid of the cassette given to us; but we did it for three-quarters of an hour here.

Second week

On the second course afternoon we did the entire body scan (three-quarters of an hour). I fell asleep a number of times. It was mentioned in discussion afterwards that the body scan is not a relaxation exercise, but an exercise in attention

[23] See his website www.aandachttraining.nl

that teaches you to be in contact with your own body. Relaxation is a by-product. Afterwards we did an exercise in seeing. We sat before a window with instructions to gaze without judgement. If we did judge we had to note this. Finally we talked about the exercises we had done at home. This week I had to continue practising the body scan, while we also had to eat the first and last mouthful of a meal with attention and note how we react to the weather.

Third week
We began by doing almost a half-hour of stretch exercises (yoga). These exercises are on side two of the first tape. This week we alternated the body scan with yoga. It is all about the attention you pay to doing the exercises. Careful, well-meaning attention helps you to get to know your body, to note your boundaries more clearly, to accept yourself as you are now, and to develop from this self-acceptance towards change. We subsequently did an exercise in order to notice the difference between focussing our gaze and allowing our gaze to open out into a broader image. We ended with an exercise for sitting in meditation. This week we did the yoga exercises at home, alternating with the body scan. We also had to observe a stress situation attentively: how do we react physically, and in our emotions and in our thoughts?

Fourth week
We did a sitting meditation exercise for up to half an hour. Different people had a lot of pain in their limbs and back. There was talk about how you could cope with this. We often want to avoid unpleasant things in our lives, run away from them. That is difficult when you're sitting so still and get pain. How do you cope with it then? Different people observed that just by remaining breathing you could bear the pain better. Others remarked that uncertainty about how long it was still going to last and the fact of having no control over it made the pain worse. Tinge said that pain is fifty percent physical, and fifty percent our reaction to it. The subject of managing your boundaries arose during the yoga exercises. It is especially important to listen to your body well, to things such as pain, blocked breathing, and palpitations. We occasionally exceed our boundaries because we have to do so much. Often we ask it of ourselves. The question also arose: how do you come to a standstill in your life, when do you get blocked? This week we had to observe what we experience during a pleasant experience. It was mainly about noticing attentively what your physical feelings are, your thoughts and your emotions, and learning to distinguish them from each other. I chose simple experiences.

Fifth week
We began our weekly session with standing yoga exercises and afterwards sitting exercises. Altogether for almost an hour. The yoga exercises were mainly

stretching exercises in different directions. During the sitting meditation we fixed our attention successively on the breath, the entire body, special bodily sensations, thoughts and finally the breath again with the entire body. We talked about it later. The intention was that you do everything with attention. Afterwards we discussed the experiences of the past week, and coping with physical tension and restlessness during the exercises. The conclusion was that you should not avoid such restlessness, but let it be by sending your breath to it with attention. There was also discussion on how to cope with the negative thoughts that come up. Apparently the point is to not identify with such feelings or thoughts, but to observe them as an attentive spectator. Tinge subsequently gave a definition of stress having to do with a relationship between a person and his environment, where there is an imbalance between ability and the burden to be borne. We talked in groups of three about what makes us stressed, how that feels and how we cope with it. A topic in the discussion afterwards was that giving attention prevents us automatically exhibiting behaviour that is damaging to ourselves in response to a specific stimulus. The attention we pay opens several options to us. I understand by this that attention helps to prevent stress, for you are better able to notice pressure signals. Furthermore, you are not obliged to revert to automatic avoidance behaviour in order to take time-out. So you deal with the situation more consciously and are therefore able to prevent stress. But how this attention may help if you are already greatly damaged, I still do not know. The attention training teaches you not to identify with your feelings and thoughts, so you can view them at a little distance; this gives you the feeling of being above them in a certain sense. Moreover, attention exercises enable you to relax. This week, we did standing yoga exercises and sitting meditation in turn. We had a whole day in Zwolle on Friday. We did yoga when prone, the body scan and the sitting meditation in the morning; in the afternoon the standing yoga, mountain meditation, walking meditation and another brief sitting body scan. We did not speak at all during this, apart from a quarter to four until almost half past four.

Sixth week

We practised a combination of standing yoga and sitting mediation during the session. Afterwards, we discussed the analysis of stress occurrences during the past week and how we had coped with them. Finally, we did various forms of walking meditation. This week we practised yoga and sitting meditation without the tapes, so in your own tempo.

Seventh week

We now did yoga and as well as sitting meditation again. Afterwards, we played communication games using walking exercises. Here we had to walk backwards while playing various roles: aggressive, passive and assertive. The intention was to experience in your body which role you usually fill automatically. By giving attention to this, you can learn to prevent yourself from habitually slipping into that role.

This week we did all the exercises with the tapes again. I could not be present for the last session and so did these exercises for two weeks. Afterwards, a personal interview with Tinge followed to round everything off.

A few conclusions and recommendations

In all the centres visited, meditation took place within a wider context of psycho-social guidance. The attention training I myself attended was complete in itself. Only the Helen Dowling Institute conducts research into the effects of guidance. This includes the course 'Living in the vortex' throughout which different forms of meditation are practiced, particularly the Kabat-Zinn programme. My conversations with those who offered or practiced meditation did not render an academically sound representation of the effects that meditation had had for those involved. But they did reaffirm the picture that had emerged from my research into the literature.

The relaxation effect is important here. Relaxation enables one to find a haven of rest in oneself, so that one can better manage the tensions accompanying sickness or pain. It is also important to train oneself in focusing attention. This makes one more aware of one's own body, thought and emotions. It leads to earlier recognition of how one reacts to stressful situations. One discerns certain mechanisms deployed to repress painful experiences more rapidly. One also learns to accept reality just as it is. Thus one acknowledges one's own limitations, not allowing oneself to be pulled over them so quickly. Because one learns to focus attention, one can give attention both to painful spots in the body and direct obsessive attention away to breathing, for example. And as one pays attention to thoughts and emotions, yet at the same time does not cling on to them, one transcends one's own thoughts and emotions to a certain extent.

That is also what the participants told me. Meditation helps them to better deal with the tensions, limitations and fears associated with their illness. They thus experience alleviation of pain and an increase in energy, or at least better regulation of it. They can also better accept their own, sometimes mutilated bodies. Moreover, meditation helps them to acquire another attitude to life, so that there is more room for a receptive attention for the benign and beautiful sides to life, including their own personality. This gives them the feeling that they are altered, enriched, have become more complete persons.

Meditation also contributes to improvement in their social relationships, in that they are more able to indicate their limitations, do not allow themselves to be overruled by demands from their social circle and can also withstand disappointing experiences in their contacts with the outside world.

Finally, meditation is revealed to have a great spiritual significance. For example, because one has learned to observe one's personal physical feelings, emotions and thoughts with relaxed attention, one learns that one is more than these thoughts and emotions. This 'transcendent' understanding is sometimes reinforced on purpose by inviting the participants to sense oneness with a greater wholeness. The latter arouses a deep response in the participants.

Meditation is not offered from a specific religious or philosophical background in any of these centres. Buddhist or Hindu elements do play a role, and Christian values too in the case of Tabor house. In general, supervisors of the meditation do not speak explicitly of spiritual objectives, in order not to frighten off participants. Almost all supervisors themselves, on further enquiry, appear to regard meditation as a spiritual discipline, and they are open to sharing spiritual experiences and questions in their course. An exception to this was Johan Tinge's attention training, which I participated in myself. There was no explicit attention paid to spirituality during the meetings. In the cassette tapes that Tinge offers for home practice there are a few careful references made to 'the greater whole' and 'life in its profundity'. Only the Helen Dowling Centre has recently considered the significance of spirituality for participants in the different forms of supervision, and is seeking a model of spirituality that can be made to operate during supervision.

The participants I interviewed had no active relationship with a church, with the exception of one woman and a couple. Yet all indicated that their illness, the way they dealt with it and the role that meditation played here had made them conscious of their relationship with the transcendent, with a spiritual reality that they called 'divine' or 'god'. Furthermore, in many cases their religious source had once again become significant, although often in another sense than before. They spoke of the sense of security in the great wholeness or of being safe with God. This realization taught them to accept their own mortality and to live with less fear. I was impressed by the openness and emotion with which they spoke of the healing power of their spiritual experiences.

I therefore conclude that meditation in the three institutions visited by me and in the attention training I participated in are offered neutrally as regards philosophy of life. Implicit and sometimes explicit spiritual values, however, sometimes pervade the supervision and the participants I spoke to had all, without exception, experienced meditation as being of great spiritual significance. In addition, I experience the definition of spirituality I chose as a useful aid to indicating the significance that meditation has for these people. Yet it struck me that the supervisors are insufficiently conscious of the spiritual grounds and implications of their supervision, in my opinion. That is why the spiritual aspects of meditation were not discussed in complete openness and insufficiently researched.

I would therefore recommend that more detailed research be done into the significance of spiritual aspects of meditation for people with physical and/or psychological symptoms. I welcome the attempts the Helen Dowling Institute makes to arrive at a good questionnaire in this field. I would recommend them to involve experts in the field of spirituality here.

I also recommend that there should be explicit religious forms of meditation for this target group. It would seem to me that neutral centres offering meditation should become more open in discussing spiritual themes implicitly offered in the practices or experienced by the participants themselves. For my research, limited as it is, demonstrates that spiritual themes and experiences mean much to the participants in these courses. Obviously I am considering Christian forms of meditation first of all here. Unfortunately I did not visit any centre where the Christian form of meditation was offered to people with physical or psychological symptoms. There is scarcely any mention of this in the literature either. I would argue that Christian centres should offer forms of Christian meditation for people with physical and/or psychological symptoms. One might expect that this would offer a resource that might mean a lot to the processing of and dealing with illness, pain, stress and the approaching end within a spiritual perspective. Meditation is a useful form of spiritual intervention for psycho-social supervision of people with cancer, but it is precisely the spiritual dimension of this intervention that is insufficiently recognized and researched. There is still much to learn in this area.

J. Bouwer

EPILOGUE
SPIRITUALITY AND MEANING IN CARE – AGENDA ITEMS FOR A CONTINUING DISCUSSION

As may be deduced from the contributions in this collection, discussion on the place and role of spirituality and meaning in healthcare may be expected to continue in the immediate future. The fact that 'general' discussion on the phenomenon of care is occurring based on diverse perspectives, strengthens the impression that this will also have ongoing effect on the field of spirituality in care. Thus the Groningen professor Post argued in his valediction that providing care is something essentially different than supplying consumer goods.[1] Here he requests attention for the conditional, social side of good care provision, with the concept of solidarity functioning as core word. The contribution of Waaijman, for example, in which he postulates the concept of 'mercy' as the heart of care, completes this vision of care. His vision rests on the fundamental reciprocity of care provision: the need of one assumes the care of the other.

If mercy and solidarity determine good and humane care, what kind of picture of humanity is assumed with this and what does this then entail for the actual practice of care? This anthology advances that man is a unity in which physical, social, psychic and spiritual aspects may be discerned. If institutions wish to offer adequate, integrated and qualitatively good care, then the care should be for the whole human being. In a provisional sense professional caregivers (i.e. nurses) should have competencies available for recognising and dealing with patients' questions of meaning; and institutions for healthcare should consider the relevance of this material for organisation and policy. Further research in this field ought to be stimulated and intensified. That was the tenor of this book.

---

1 D. Post, *Een spannende toekomst voor zorg en zekerheid* (An exciting future for care and certainty), Houten-Mechelen: Bohn Stafleu Van Loghum, 2003, 15. Post, em. Professor in social medicine, refers here in his farewell lecture (13th May, 2003) to Hattinga Verschure's analysis of the care concept. He argues that care is based on social motives amongst which solidarity is a key concept. People do not choose voluntarily for being cared for. It is from a necessity due to illness or impairment.

The question is rather which aspects of the discussion on spirituality and meaning in healthcare should or will determine the agenda in the future. It can be concluded from the contributions in this collection that this discussion takes place explicitly or implicitly on five levels, namely the fundamental-substantiated, organisational-institutional, professional, socio-cultural and empirical-scientific levels. As an epilogue I will now briefly attempt to work out the most important discussion points on the five levels mentioned.

1. Fundamental substantiation

It is not only apparent from the contributions in this collection, but also from other sources, that no consensus exists regarding conceptualising the concept of care – and along with this also the concept of spirituality.[2] One person defines spirituality in religious terms, while another argues that spirituality is a quality that rises above religious affiliation whereby an important given is the attempt of the individual for inspiration, wonderment, meaning and goal in life. Persons who do not believe in a (personal) God, or do not believe in a God at all, are also spiritual beings. A philosophic-anthropological conceptualisation of the term spirituality can reckon on a broader basis for this discussion in healthcare. Accordingly, a strict association with religion will have to be avoided if one wishes to come to generalising conclusions. This does not alter the fact that one can consciously choose to research the relationship between religion and health, or between Christian and Islamic spirituality, for example, and health. Or the influence that the aforementioned philosophies of life that the patient may have, exerts on the illness and possibly on the healing process. Conceptualisation is an important agenda point for discussion in the future, whereby the connection and the differentiation of spirituality to and from meaning, religion and philosophy of life will have to be demonstrated.

2. Institutional implementation

Holistic care provision also assumes an institution for healthcare which has reflected on the implications of spirituality for organisation and policy at the

---

[2] C.G. Ellison & J.S. Levin, 'The religion-health connection: Evidence, theory and future directions', in: *Health Education & Behavior* 25 (1998) no 6, 700-720. See also W. Carr, 'Some reflections on spirituality; religion and mental health', in: *Mental Health, Religion and Culture* 3 (2000) no 1, 1-12; B. Carroll, 'A phenomenological exploration of the nature of spirituality and spiritual care', in: *Mortality* 6 (2001) no 1, 81-99; M.J. Mahoney & G.M. Graci, 'The meanings and correlates of spirituality: Suggestions from an exploratory survey of experts', in: *Death Studies* 23 (1999) no 6, 521-529.

pro-active and strategic level. More expressly than ever before, institutions will have to ask themselves how the life philosophies of the care seekers are bound up with the quality of care offered. But institutions will also have to ask themselves what the notion of spirituality implies for the institution as employer. Aspects such as identity, vision, and mission – as is evident from Gribnau, Pijnenburg and Bakker's contributions – ought to remain fixed items on the agenda in the future. For the interaction between care seeker and caregiver, or care provider takes place on the meso level (within one's own bosom). There will have to be reflection on the notion of 'the spiritual organisation' on account of this interactive moment or this structure. Here the identification of the internal aspects of material or perceptible manifestations of power is involved.[3] Organisations have a 'personality, a character, an inner disposition and an ethos analogous to (but separate from) the persons who constitute them.[4] What do not only care seekers, but also caregivers get from this 'person'? Are the treatment, appreciation, labour conditions and organisation culture such that employees can develop themselves as caregivers?

3. Professional care providers

A following point on the agenda requiring reflection and discussion, is the question of demarcating the responsibilities of caregivers where the care seekers' spirituality is concerned. The spiritual caregiver – a valuable and recognised discipline within health care – is charged with the guidance of and aid to people in giving meaning to their existence in the face of illness, suffering, invalidity and death. Therefore it is best to arrive at a clear demarcation of the provinces of the diverse disciplines. It would be very easy to transgress an ethical and professional boundary here. The spiritual caregiver is concerned with the ultimate or ontological meaning of the individual, as distinct from everyday meaning making. Questions on the why of suffering, correct action in this context and the expectations that one may or be allowed to cherish regarding the future, form part of the domain that we may dub 'holy'. They assume a connection to an external reality, an ideal, a unity of meaning, a framework of life, something that transcends the individual. Not everyone who forms his/her philosophy of life with integrity and awareness can call him/herself an expert in the field of the functioning of the spirit in relation to ultimate meaning. Training is necessary. And

---

3 D. Lyall, 'Spiritual institutions?', in: H. Orchard (Ed.), *Spirituality in health care contexts*, London: Kingsley, 2001, 52.

4 Ibidem.

according to the Individual Health Care Professions Act[5], not being competent makes a person not qualified.

Reflection on this point will therefore also have to focus on the training and further training or education necessary for dealing with questions concerning the giving of meaning. This particularly applies to those caring professions directly involved with care seekers, such as nurses, doctors, those doing social work and psychologists. One could think here of knowledge gained over diverse philosophic traditions and diagnostic skills in the field of spirituality. Holistic care also assumes good co-operation between the diverse disciplines and a well coordinated culture of inter-referral. Training and further education is an important factor in complying with this condition.

4. Socio-cultural context

This point is indirectly connected to the previous one. The discussion on spirituality in health care cannot be conducted without reflecting on the context in which the care must be given. Dutch society is characterised on the one hand by concepts such as individualism and post modernism, but on the other hand by concepts such as multiculturalism and pluralism. Caregivers and care providers will therefore have to be aware of the fact that concepts of care have not only nestled down in the heads of policy makers, but also in the heads of care seekers, who are birds of all kinds of philosophic feathers. How does this connect to people's concept of illness? What link is there to the people's convictions? This means that care providers must also be able to deal with the desires, needs and expectations – and thus also the spirituality – of people coming from other traditions than those of the Dutch. For the new maxim is: 'the patient is central'. This statement in its turn gives rise to questions as to the implications it has for the identity, integration and manner of working of the spiritual caregiver. For the caregiver is set against the background of article 3 of the Quality Act, in which it is determined that patients have the right to the spiritual care 'that suits them'. Finally, a question on the meta level: what does the multicultural context mean – as a framework in which care for spirituality takes place – for Post's statement that there must be a greater emphasis on the social character of the Dutch care system in the future.[6] For a humane and sympathetic care system will not allow the market to take its course without restraint.

---

5 In Dutch: the BIG Act.

6 Post, *Een spannende toekomst*, 39.

5. Empirical-scientific research

Spirituality as phenomenon is difficult to research, due to its subjective nature and poly-interpretability. This statement increases the topicality of the earlier indicated necessity for a simple conceptualising of spirituality. This will also serve to put that term into operation for empirical research. Only the question is: what method will serve research in the field of spirituality and meaning the best? At the moment, there is ongoing discussion as to whether spirituality may or must be researched qualitatively or quantitatively. Some argue for a combination of these two methods, because they can compliment each other.[7] However that may be: in the future, research must be started into the development of measuring instruments to obtain more insight into the relationship between spirituality, health and care. For the time being, exploratory and descriptive qualitative research may clear the way to this.[8] Because this is undeveloped ground, research can be initiated into the possibility of effect studies, interaction research, methodological implications such as type research, design, samples and analysis techniques. And it can also be initiated into the influence of the spirituality of the care provider on the provision of care, and the influence of the care seeker's spirituality on the illness and the healing process.

These points call up the image of an exciting adventure in an environment in which philosophy of life and religion as factors to be taken into account in care are no longer self-evident, and talk of spirituality and meaning has only just begun. The future will show whether this material will find its way into the organisation, policy and actual practice of care. It is worth taking the trouble to enter into this discussion and to continue it. For humanity is at stake.

---

7 L.J. Tiesinga, J. Bouwer, H. Jochemsen, H. Blommenstijn, K. Waaijman & D. Post, 'Spiritualiteit: (on)gezondheid en zorg; een aanwezige en onderzoekbare relatie?' (Spirituality, health, illness and care: a present and researchable relationship?), in: *Tijdschrift voor Gezondheidswetenschappen* (Journal for Health Sciences) 80 (2002) no 8, 537.

8 Ibidem.

Appendix 1:

WORKING GROUP RESEARCH IN THE FIELD OF SPIRITUALITY-HEALTH-CARE (RESPIRE)

RESPIRE
The working group RESPIRE is composed of field researchers into questions concerning spirituality in the area of health care. RESPIRE wishes to contribute to the integration of spirituality, health and care.

Aims
1. To give more publicity to the theme spirituality-health-care;
2. Form theory in the area of spirituality-health-care;
3. Stimulate research;
4. Further the implementation of theory into practice, in the field of spirituality-health-care

Procedure
1. Discuss research results;
2. Coordinate research plans and proposals;
3. Agreements on use of measuring instruments;
4. Where possible and wise, promote co-operation

Results
1. Organising symposia;
2. Writing articles, including those for forums

Structure
RESPIRE consists of the following persons: Prof. Dr D. Post, Prof. Dr. H. Jochemsen, Prof. Dr J. Bouwer, Prof. Dr. K. Waaijman, Prof. Dr. H. Blommestijn en Dr, L.J. Tiesinga.

Information
For more detailed information please contact Dr L.J. Tiesinga, Rijksuniversiteit Groningen, Faculty of Medical Sciences, Discipline group Health Sciences, Department Care Sciences, P.O. Box 196, 9700 AD Groningen, The Netherlands, email: L.J.Tiesinga@med.rug.nl

Appendix 2:

FAITH AND PHILOSOPHY OF LIFE FOUNDATION

The Faith and Philosophy of Life Foundation was established to promote attention to the element of philosophy of life within care among management and those working in homecare. The fusion between the National Home Nursing Service and the Central Council for Family Care Foundation in 1990 gave birth to the National Association for Homecare. This signified a broadening of the target group for the Foundation, in that family carers now were seen as being included. Since then the target group has consisted of those working in home care in the broad sense of the word and therefore includes: district nurses, district orderlies and home helps.

Aim

The Foundation has as its aim:

- The recognition of faith and philosophy of life as a function of health care. It indicate that it wishes to heed the questions of meaning that people wrestle with. These questions are often posed in the course of coming to terms with the illness or aging process of the client.
- Education in philosophy of life for those working in homecare by helping them to look out for the personal questions and problems which a person in homecare struggles with.
- Offering insight through conveying knowledge to workers in homecare about what faith and philosophy of life can mean to a person in difficult situations.

Implementation

The Foundation intends to achieve its aims through giving subsidies for equipment days, maintaining contacts with regional project groups, supporting project groups for considering the theme of philosophy of life in homecare and publishing brochures about themes in this field.

Information

National Association for Home Care
P.O. Box 100
3980 CC Bunnik
The Netherlands
Tel: +31-30-6596211

Appendix 3:

PROTESTANT THEOLOGICAL UNIVERSITY KAMPEN AND HEALTHCARE

It has recently become possible to take a course of studies on spiritual care in healthcare at the Protestant Theological University Kampen. The University offers two Masters degrees in this area:

1. The Masters degree Man and Care (Master of Spiritual Care). Length of study is one year full time or eighteen months part time after obtaining a recognised Bachelor Theology Plus or a transitional Bachelor Theology Plus after a HBO (Higher Professional Education) Bachelor. It is a theoretical course of studies, particularly interesting for people who are active in health care as clerical or pastoral workers.
2. The Master degree Spiritual Care (Master of Theology and Spiritual Care). This variant has been approved by the Protestant Church in the Netherlands as being a study leading to obtaining the qualification of ministry within this church. The length of study is three years after obtaining a recognised Bachelor of Theology Classical.

Subjects of the study programme
A selection of subjects that are optional or compulsory in various courses:
- Introduction to context and work areas of spiritual care
- Introduction to spiritual care
- Practice investigation
- Philosophical anthropology
- The interview in the helping professions
- Literature and sickness
- Religion and contingency (about life, sickness, health and death in the great religions)
- Person, meaning-making and coping
- Philosophy of life diagnostics, agogics (social science relating to the promotion of personal, social and cultural welfare) and didactics
- Medical and care ethics (including dilemmas in health and care ethics)
- Masters thesis
- Practical sections (For Master of Spiritual Care)

Information
For more information about intake requirements and the like:
Please request a folder via +31 38 337 1614 or via info@pthu.nl
Or visit the university website: www.pthu.nl

PERSONALIA

Dr D.J. BAKKER is (emeritus) Medical Director of the Academic Medical Centre, Amsterdam, surgeon N.P. and Member of the Board of Hospice Curia

Prof Dr J. BOUWER was University Senior Lecturer and Extraordinary Professor of Spiritual Care in Health Care Institutions at the Protestant Theological University in Kampen and is Professor of Coaching Science and Meaning at the Alba-University in Veldhoven

Dr K.E. BRAS was University Lecturer in Spirituality at the Theological University Kampen and is Congregation minister of the Protestant Church in the Netherlands in Gorinchem

Dr B.S. CUSVELLER is a nurse, philosopher and lecturer associated with the Prof Dr G.A. Lindeboom Institute, Ede

Prof Dr F.W.J. GRIBNAU was a member of the Board of Directors of the UMC St Radboud, Nijmegen, internist N.P, and is emeritus Professor of Clinical Pharmacology at the Faculty of Medical Science at the same university

Prof Dr H. JOCHEMSEN is Director of the Prof Dr G.A. Lindeboom Institute, Ede and Extraordinary Professor of Medical Ethics at the Free University, Amsterdam

Drs M. KLAASE-CARPENTIER was involved in the Prof Dr G.A. Lindeboom Institute, Ede as a researcher on project basis

Drs M.A.M. PIJNENBURG is a staff member on the department of Ethics, Philosophy and History of Medicine at the UMC St Radboud, Nijmegen

Drs A. van de SCHEUR was a researcher at the Prof Dr G.A. Lindeboom Institute, Ede. At present, she is Assistant Research Fellow at the University of Maastricht

Dr L.J. TIESINGA is University Lecturer in Health Sciences at the Faculty of Medical Sciences at the University of Groningen

Prof Dr K. WAAIJMAN is Director of the Titus Brandsma Institute and emeritus Professor of Spirituality at the Radboud University, Nijmegen

Studies in Spirituality Supplements

2. **Franco Imoda**, *Human Development. Psychology and Mystery*, 1998, 397 p., ISBN: 90-429-0028-8.

3. **Marieke van Baest**, *Poetry of Hadewijch*, 1998, VIII-330 p., ISBN: 90-429-0668-7.

4. **Hildegard Elisabeth Keller**, *My Secret is Mine. Studies on Religion and Eros in the German Middle Ages*, 2000, VIII-294 p., ISBN: 90-429-0871-8.

5. **Franco Imoda**, *A Journey to Freedom. An Interdisciplinary Approach to the Anthropology of Formation*, 2000, XIV-482 p., ISBN: 90-429-0894-7.

6. **Albrecht Classen**, *'Mein Seel fang an zu singen'. Religiöse Frauenlieder des 15.-16. Jahrhunderts. Kritische Studien und Textedition*, 2002, 395 p., ISBN: 90-429-1098-4.

7. **Marie L. Baird**, *On the Side of the Angels. Ethics and Post-Holocaust Spirituality*, 2002, 143 p., ISBN: 90-429-1156-5.

8. **Kees Waaijman**, *Spirituality. Forms, Foundations, Methods*, 2002, VIII-968 p., ISBN: 90-429-1183-2.

9. **John D. Green**, *'A Strange Tongue'. Tradition, Language and the Appropriation of Mystical Experiences in the Late Fourteenth-Century England and Sixteenth-Century Spain*, 2002, VII-227 p., ISBN: 90-429-1236-7.

10. **Hein Blommestijn, Charles Caspers and Rijcklof Hofman (Eds.)**, *Spirituality Renewed. Studies on Significant Representatives of the Modern Devotion*, 2003, VI-276 p., ISBN: 90-429-1327-4.

11. **Donald J. Moores**, *Mystical Discourse in Wordsworth and Whitman. A Transatlantic Bridge*, 2006, VII-286 p., ISBN: 90-429-1809-8.

12. **Alessandro Manenti, Stefano Guarinelli and Hans Zollner (Eds.)**, *Formation and the Person. Essays in Theory and Practice*, 2007, VIII-303 p., ISBN 978-90-429-1881-8.

13. **Elisabeth Hense**, *Die Kammer der Andacht. Formbeschreibung einer Theaterproduktion*, 2007, X-114 p., ISBN 978-90-429-1966-2.

14. **John D. Green**, *'Augustinianism'. Studies in the Process of Spiritual Transvaluation,* 2007, VIII-114 p., ISBN 978-90-429-1976-1.

15. **Una Agnew, Bernadette Flanagan and Greg Heylin (Eds.)**, *'With Wisdom Seeking God'. The Academic Study of Spirituality*, 2008, X-282 p., ISBN 978-90-429-2030-9.

16. **Edy Korthals Altes**, *'Spiritual awakening'. The Hidden Key to Peace and Security, Just and Sustainable Economics, A Responsible European Union*, 2008, VIII-238 p., ISBN 978-90-429-2046-0.

PRINTED ON PERMANENT PAPER • IMPRIME SUR PAPIER PERMANENT • GEDRUKT OP DUURZAAM PAPIER - ISO 9706

N.V. PEETERS S.A., WAROTSTRAAT 50, B-3020 HERENT